SEX
games

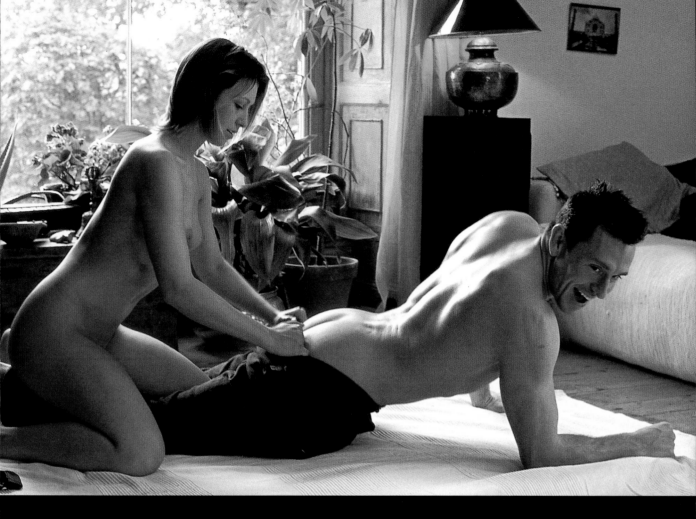

SEX
games

Linda Sonntag

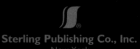

Sterling Publishing Co., Inc.
New York

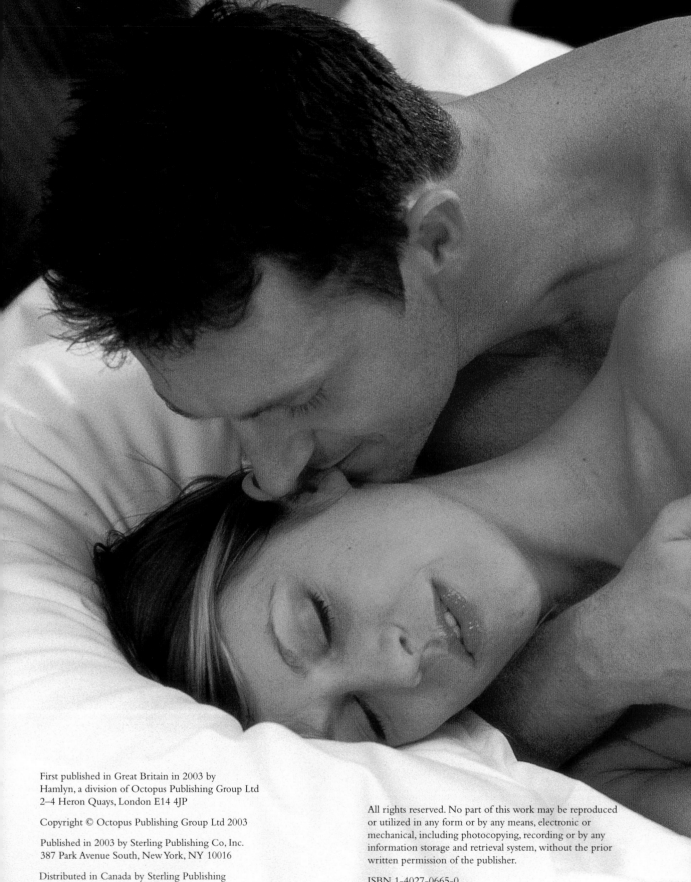

First published in Great Britain in 2003 by
Hamlyn, a division of Octopus Publishing Group Ltd
2–4 Heron Quays, London E14 4JP

Copyright © Octopus Publishing Group Ltd 2003

Published in 2003 by Sterling Publishing Co, Inc.
387 Park Avenue South, New York, NY 10016

Distributed in Canada by Sterling Publishing
165 Dufferin Street, Toronto, Ontario M6K 3H67, Canada.

Library of Congress Cataloging-in-Publication Data Available

ISBN 1-4027-0665-0

Printed in Hong Kong

10 9 8 7 6 5 4 3

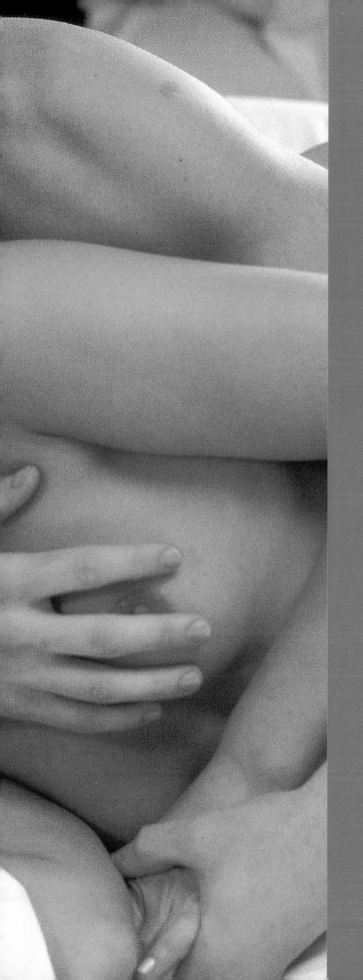

Contents

WARNING With the prevalence of AIDS and other sexually transmitted diseases, if you do not practise safe sex you are risking your life and your partner's life.

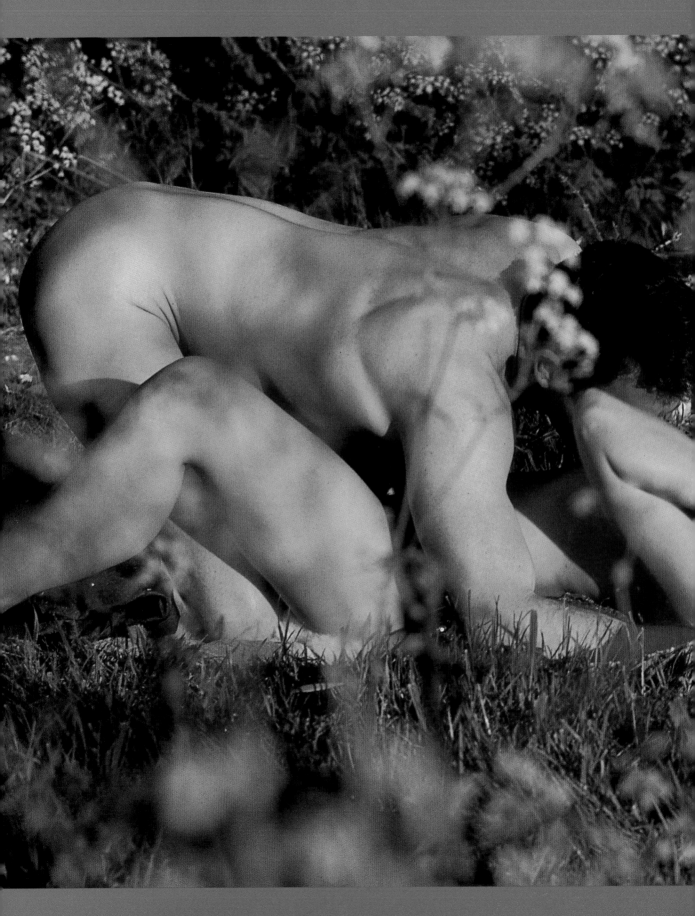

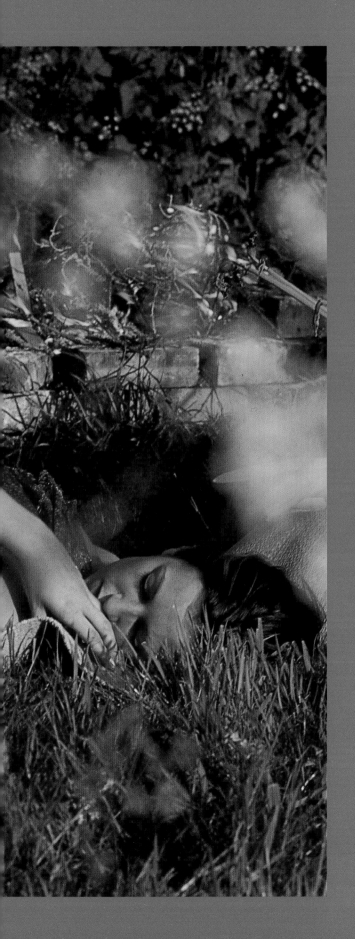

Introduction

Are you ready to explore your sexuality and have the most fun ever in bed? Do you long to discover ways of pleasing your partner that will dissolve all inhibitions? Sometimes the furious pace of living in the 21st century makes it difficult to remember that sex is about play – when the rest of life is goal-orientated it's all too easy to start thinking about what you do in bed in terms of achievements.

Do you take the anxieties and pressures of your daily life to bed with you? Have you lost the knack of laughing in bed? Have you forgotten how to make love anywhere else? This book will show you how to take the stress out of sex and learn new ways of relaxing together. Slowly and deliciously, you can explore imaginative and erotic touching and enjoy a superb whole-body sensual massage. If your sex life has got stuck in a rut and become a no-frills fast track to orgasm, you'll find plenty of ideas for spicing things up and lots of ways of rediscovering your own sensuality and sense of fun – and that of the person you fell in love with. And of course if you're passionate about your lover and don't want the magic to fade, you can learn some simple, stunningly effective new techniques – sex moves designed to drive your partner wild, tricks to make a man last longer and a woman come more quickly.

Then there are sexy extracts to read in bed, raunchy ideas for a toy box full of naughty novelties and some unusual ways of letting rip with fantasy. So cuddle up with your beloved and get reading…

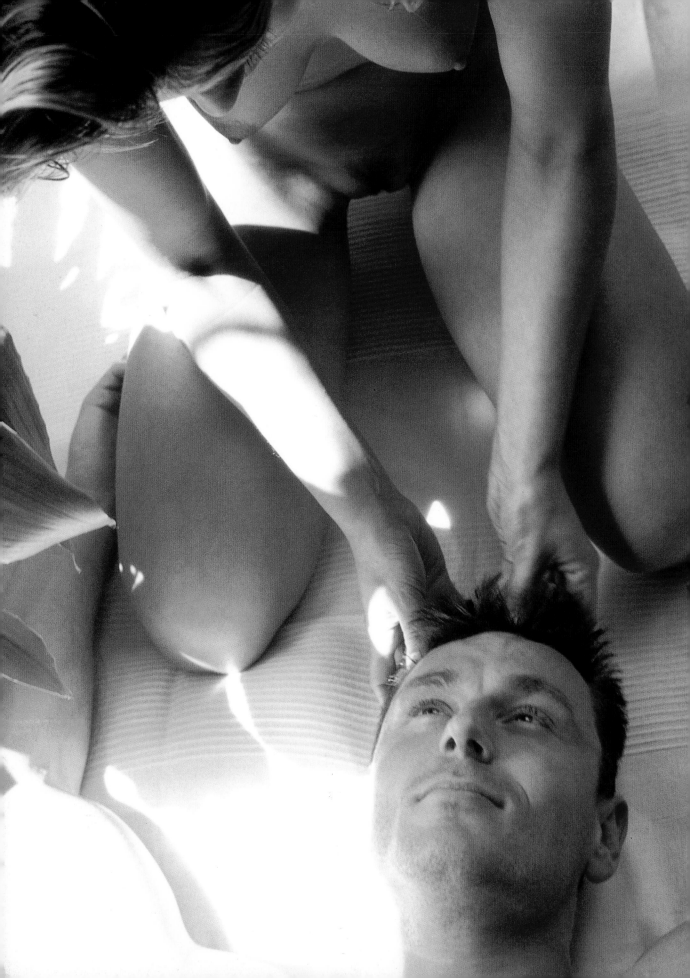

WARM UP FOR SEX

This erotic massage sequence is full of surprises that open the door to total body sensation. It isn't targeted on the obvious erogenous zones, but treats all of the body equally, allowing you to discover parts of each other that you may never have explored before – such as the scalp, the backs of the knees and the feet. When your partner expects your hands to linger on her breasts and you skim smoothly on, you build up erotic anticipation and pass the intense, alive feelings to the next part that you touch, until her whole body becomes a finely tuned pleasure zone. Don't talk, don't think, just feel...

The power of touch

Touch is the most intimate form of communication and massage is the oldest and most instinctive form of healing. Giving your partner a really loving massage signifies total acceptance of his (or her) body. It transmits affirmation and boosts self-esteem. At its best, a massage will touch his emotions as much as it touches his body. It will help to get rid of mental and physical stress and thereby enable him to centre himself inside sensation, shutting out all distractions in the process.

Massage can help

These are the symptoms of stress to look out for in your partner:

Looking dishevelled and exhausted

Feeling that clothing and shoes are uncomfortable and too tight

Continual stretching and rubbing to ease aches and pains in shoulders, neck and back

Being argumentative and frustrated, and aggressively repeating parts of unfulfilling conversations that occurred during the day

Being clumsy, accident-prone and unable to concentrate

Having a short fuse with nearest and dearest, and being intolerant of small inconveniences

Negative body language – continual pacing and impatient repetitive actions such as tapping feet or drumming fingers

Bad sitting posture – either wound up with one leg twined around the other, or completely slumped

Time to Unwind

After a day at work, sitting for long periods as well as the inevitable stress of schedules, deadlines and personality clashes, your partner is probably suffering aches and pains, aggression and frustration. Massage can ease tension and eliminate toxins from his body tissues. Once he is fully relaxed you can turn your attention to his erogenous zones. However, don't use massage as a way of manipulating his feelings and trying to persuade him to have sex if he's not ready for it.

The gentle approach

Don't offer alcohol, tobacco or other drugs – they will act first as an accelerator, increasing the outpouring of negativity, then gradually numb and depress the feelings – which won't make for a relaxing evening or good sex later.

Listen. Empathize. Don't offer solutions – they will be rejected and you'll find yourself catapulted into an argument.

When your partner has calmed down sufficiently and is sitting down, begin a gentle massage of the back of the neck and shoulders. If you get a good reaction, suggest a full massage for later.

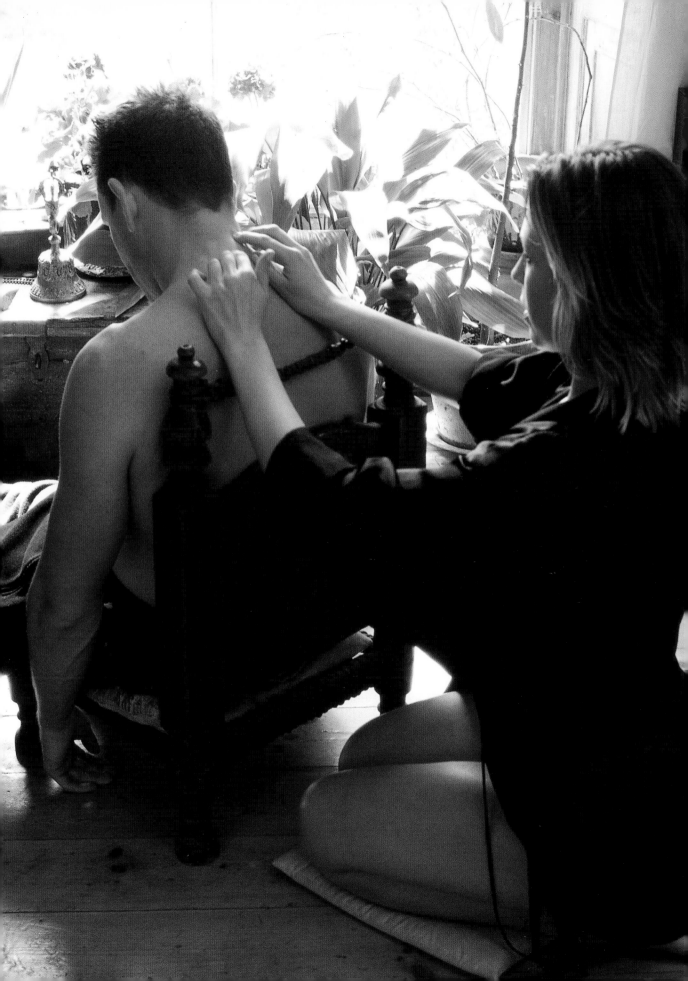

Handwork 1

The laying on of hands is comforting, reassuring, calming and healing. In addition, you will need to learn four basic massage strokes: gliding, kneading, deep pressure and percussion.

Technique 1: Gliding

Let your hands glide smoothly and rhythmically over your partner's skin. The soothing nature of this stroke makes it ideal for starting and finishing a session – use a broad stroke to 'join up' the body after having worked on specific areas.

1. Vary the firmness and speed of your strokes, and experiment with applying most pressure from the heel of your hand, the palms or the fingertips.

2. Try drawing wavy lines on your partner's skin, opening out your fingers and closing them again.

3. Try very light pressure with fingertips only. This is quite difficult to do without tickling, so wait until your partner is fully relaxed.

4. Use alternate strokes – let one hand follow the other, skimming across your partner's skin as if you were brushing crumbs towards yourself.

5. Make big circles with your hands, letting one hand follow the other. This is a very good stroke for centring the body and banishing mental stress.

6. From a kneeling position at your partner's head, glide both your hands down her back together, pushing quite firmly, then draw them up again.

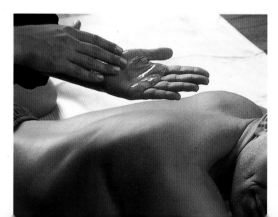

Massage tips

Remove jewellery and make sure nails are short and smooth.

Make sure the room is warm enough. Professional masseurs cover the part of the body that they are not working on with a light blanket – you could try a sensuous silk scarf instead.

Use massage oil to lubricate your partner's skin. Choose a fragrance you both like.

Warm your chosen massage oil between the palms of your hands before you apply it – don't pour it on to your partner's skin directly from the bottle as this will startle him and break the mood.

Keep contact with at least one hand on the body as you change position, and if you have to break contact, do so gently, and begin again lightly.

Don't encourage conversation while you massage – the idea is to let daily life float away from you. But don't be surprised if deeply felt sentiments are voiced out of the blue.

Why massage is good for sex

- Massage puts you in touch with a deeper sense of self
- It's a relaxing way of tuning into each other without words
- It allows time and space for simply being together
- It allows you to observe your partner's body and responses
- It allows intuition to take over
- There is no pressure to perform

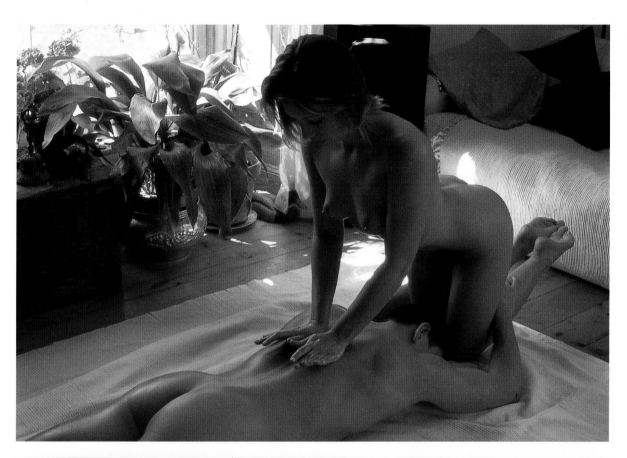

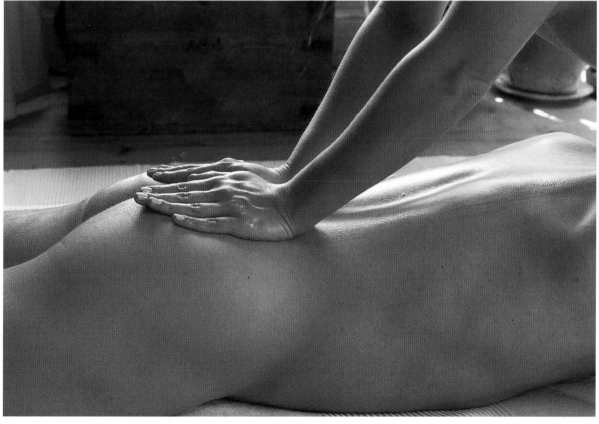

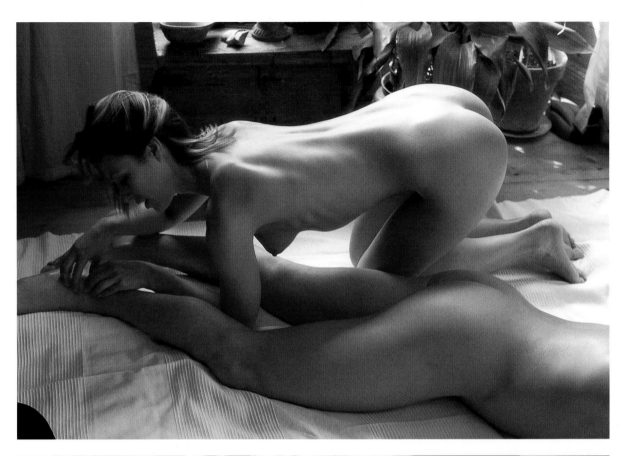

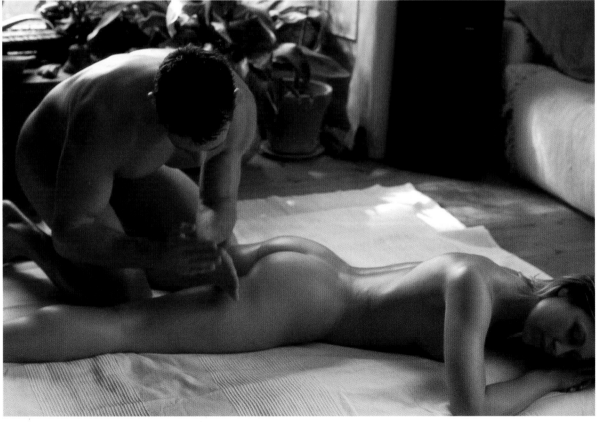

Handwork 2

Technique 2: Kneading

A vigorous stroke that gives instant relief, transforming the body under your hands from sluggish and fatigued to light and energetic. The key lies in rhythmic repetition, building up a momentum that is almost hypnotic.

Choose a fleshy area on which to practise, such as the buttocks. Put your palms flat on your partner's body with fingers together and your hands pointing at 45° towards each other. Make small circles with your hands, moving them up and outwards in turn, following each other. Now add the thumb movement – every time your hand moves up and out, your thumb moves separately behind it, grasping the flesh and pushing it firmly along, as if you were kneading bread. Feel tensed muscles softening under your hands as you work.

A variation on this stroke is wringing, where the hands work simultaneously in opposite directions. Another is pulling. Sitting on one side of your partner, reach across to the other side of her back and pull the flesh firmly towards you with alternate hands. A third variation is to nip the flesh between fingers and thumb, tugging and then releasing. Use alternate hands.

Technique 3: Deep pressure

Use your thumbs to apply deep pressure, but wait until your partner is fully relaxed, or it might hurt. Press firmly into the flesh with the balls of your thumbs, making little circles and pushing the skin away from you. Put your weight behind the movement. Work with both thumbs together or use them alternately, moving across areas of particular tension to disperse knots and toxins.

Technique 4: Percussion

These are strong rhythmic movements that quickly get right through the defences your partner has been building up during the working day. Invigorating rather than sensual, this is a stroke to use on fleshy parts of the body to get your partner relaxed for later on. In percussion, always allow the hand to relax at the wrist before contact so that you are using the weight of your hand rather than the force of your whole arm. Keep up a strong hypnotic rhythm – think of the steady drumming of heavy rain.

One-handed percussion: as your left hand glides over your partner's skin, pound it repeatedly with the weight of your right fist.

Two-handed percussion: keep up a loose drumming rhythm, working with alternate fists. Work lightly on sensitive areas, trying percussion with the tips of your index fingers.

Hacking: work with palms facing each other, hands flat, fingers together. This is good on the buttocks, thighs and calves, but could be painful elsewhere.

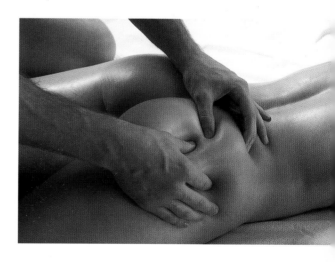

The back

The expressions 'pain in the neck', 'I took it in the neck' and 'it really got my back up' say everything about the body's major stress sites. The back and the neck have everything to do with how we hold ourselves – and how we protect and defend ourselves from the rest of the world. The more problems in our lives, the greater the tension in these key areas. Stress and fear are the enemies of sex, so the first thing you need to do for a stressed-out partner is rub her back. Here's how to do it properly to release those hard knots of tension that are ruining her mood.

Sexual stress buster 1

1. Kneel astride your partner's buttocks for warm intimate contact. Begin by leaning forwards and working on the base of the neck with firm pressure and small deep kneading strokes with the thumbs and fingers. Really lose yourself, allowing the knots of tension to dictate your movements.

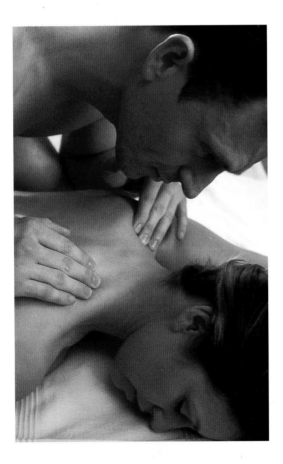

Try to become invisible, existing only in the intuitive movements of your hands.

2. Move to your partner's side so that you can work the shoulder nearest you. Using fine and detailed pressure with the fingers and thumbs, feel your way round the contours of the shoulder blade, smoothing out any grittiness as you go. Lift the shoulder and rotate it, continuing to work the flesh with the other hand. Repeat on the other shoulder.

3. Straddle your partner again and work up and down the back with broad gliding strokes, pushing the flesh towards the neck under your hands, then dragging your palms back down with splayed fingers trailing.

4. Repeat several times, then work a thumb's width down either side of the spine, using walking steps with your fingers and thumbs and wiggling them in minute circles where they land. Don't touch your partner's spine, as contact here can be uncomfortable.

5. Finish the back massage with broad sensual gliding stokes that go up the centre of the back and sweep down the sides.

6. Straddling your partner's legs without putting pressure on them, move on to the buttocks. Use vigorous kneading strokes, or try pulling and releasing, pummelling, hacking and nipping. Push the soft flesh up towards the back and outwards – stretching movements that stimulate the genital area without touching it.

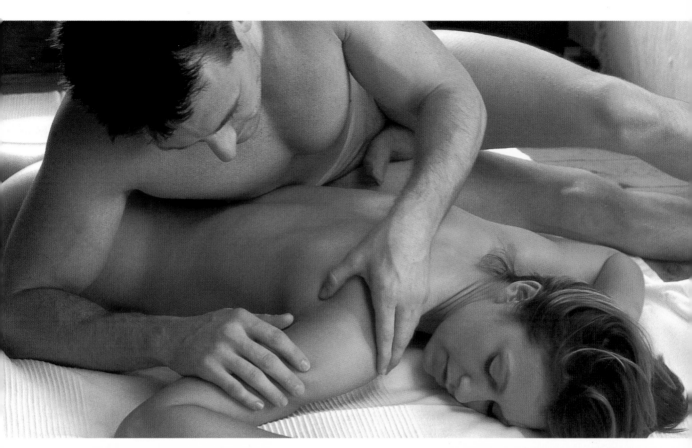

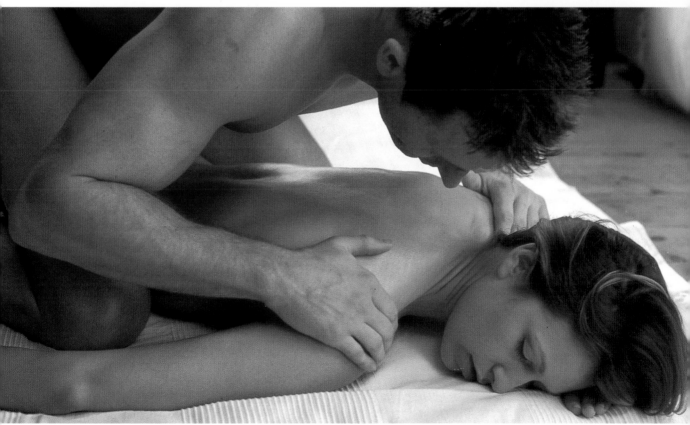

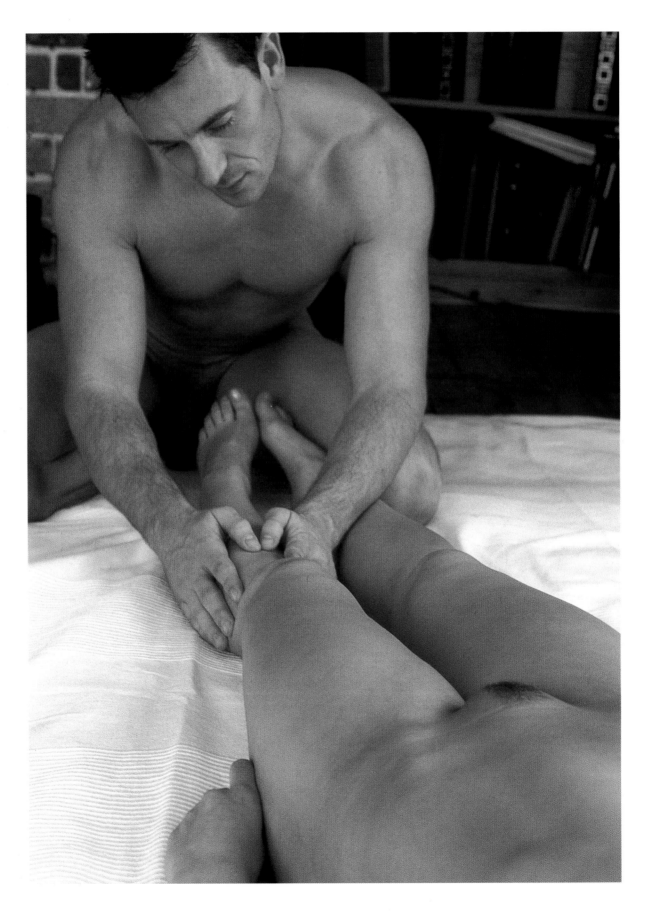

Legs and arms

One of the great benefits of erotic massage is the feeling it gives of being cherished all over. Yet some parts of the body get badly neglected – how often, for example, do you touch or caress your partner's lower legs or feet? It may be that no one has paid any loving attention to these extremities since your partner was little. Studying her limbs in detail as you stroke them to learn their contours and feel the flesh and muscles respond under your touch can give your partner a blissful feeling of security and belonging. Having every part of her body attended to will give her a zinging feeling of being really alive, which in turn makes for lively, super-sensitive sex.

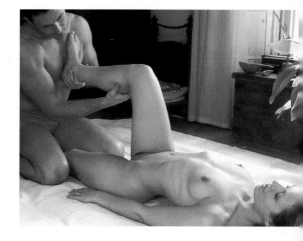

Sexual tension buster 2

Get the circulation going and the blood oxygenated by working the legs and arms towards the heart.

1. With your partner lying on her back, start at the ankles. Wrap your hands around them, making close contact with your palms and fingers against her skin. With all circulation strokes, the idea is to move the hands together, pushing the blood in the direction of the heart. Work up the legs, and as you come back down again, keep the pressure in the same direction, towards the heart.

2. Now work the arms in the same way, again with the strokes in the direction of the heart.

And while you're there...

With your partner lying on her back, raise her lower leg to make a right angle with the floor. Lean forwards and rest the sole of her foot on your chest. Wrap your hands round the calf and massage it deeply towards the heart, applying little circles of pressure with your thumbs.

Massage your partner's inner thighs with deep thumb pressure. Work up to the genitals but don't touch them. An invigorating massage will get the blood pumping in the genital area.

Focus on the knee

Next it's the turn of the knees, another erotically sensitive and much neglected part of the body. The knee is the body's most complicated joint. Its smooth movement is hampered by tension in the muscles above and below it. You have already released this tension, so now you can give your partner a pleasure that he may never have experienced before by working on the knee itself.

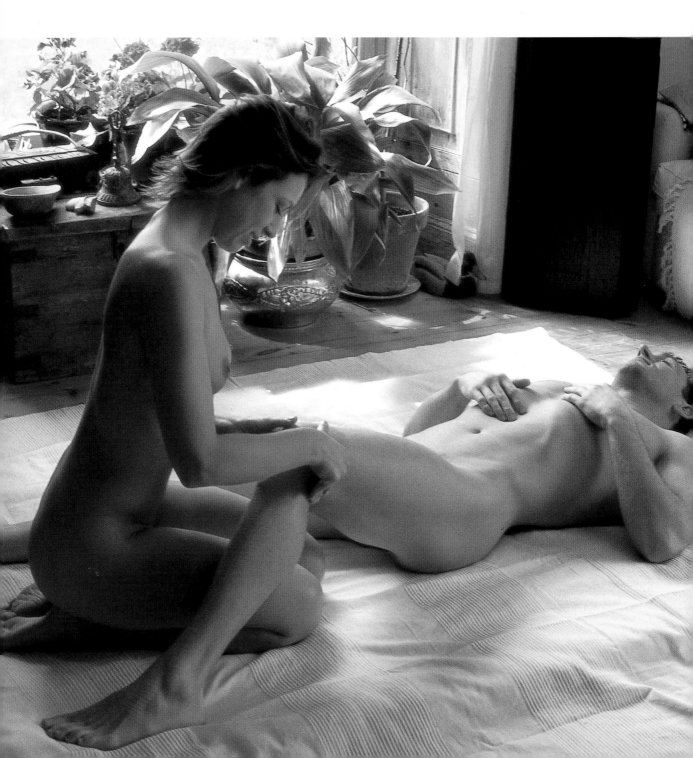

And while you're there...

Position yourself just below your partner's hips. Raise the leg nearest you, supporting it with one hand clasping the calf and the other under the thigh. Then, still holding the calf, place the palm of your other hand on the front of his leg just below his knee and push forwards with your body weight, so that his leg bends at the knee, his knee moves towards his chest, and his heel touches his thigh.

Stop as soon as you feel resistance – don't force the leg, as this could be painful.

Repeat, stretching the leg out and folding it towards his body five times. You should feel him relax a little more each time.

Do the same with the other leg. This exercise is very expansive and gives a great sensation of freedom and openness. Use this move to indirectly stimulate and improve blood supply to the genital area.

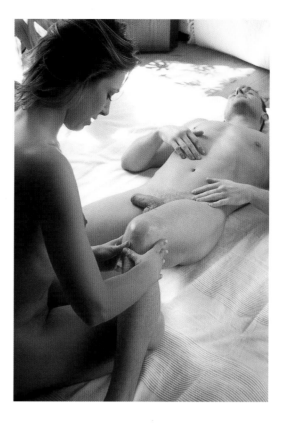

Sexual tension buster 3

1. With your partner lying on his back, work on the fronts of his legs from the ankles to the tops of the thighs. Begin with generous gliding strokes up and down the outsides of the legs to warm him and connect him top to bottom.

2. Then knead with gentle pressure either side of the shin. Work more vigorously on the thighs, kneading thoroughly until his flesh feels warm and tingling with life.

3. Sitting alongside the lower leg, raise his knee slightly from the floor, taking its weight in both hands. With your fingers under the knee and your thumbs above it, brush your thumbs repeatedly over the kneecap. Use the lightest of strokes, as any pressure here would be uncomfortable.

4. Now use your thumbs to work very gently in the groove below the kneecap, meanwhile stroking your fingers in and around the crease at the fleshy back of the knee. Avoid pressing against the tendons. As you build up speed you and your partner will feel a pleasant relaxing warmth gathering in the area.

Up and down to the feet

Worries about sex, whatever their nature, cause tension to build up in the legs. Sometimes this leads to excruciating cramps in the calf muscles, which tend to strike during the small hours of the morning. Practise this move as part of your erotic massage to keep the legs relaxed and supple.

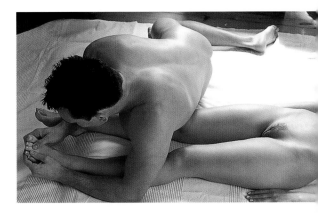

Sexual tension buster 4

Forearm compression causes warm pleasant feelings to travel up and down your partner's leg. Oil your forearm first to make it glide more smoothly across her leg – the more body hair there is at the point of contact, the more oil you will need to use.

1. Lift your partner's leg from the floor with both hands and hold it by the ankle so that the knee is comfortably raised. Clench your fist to tighten the muscles in your arm, then press the inside of your forearm against her calf, just above the ankle. Pulling all the while towards your body, move your arm up towards her knee, rotating it as if you were polishing her leg.

2. When you get to the knee, lean forwards and work on the upper side of her thigh, bearing down with your weight and continuing to 'polish' to the top of her thigh.

3. Repeat several times then lower her leg to the floor using both hands and move on to do the same to the other leg.

And while you're there...

Try this with the feet. Sit facing the tops of her feet with your back towards her face. Holding one foot in both hands, work delicately with your thumbs, feeling around all the bones of the feet from the base of the toes up towards the ankle. Be careful not to spoil the mood by inadvertently tickling your partner with a feathery touch on her soles.

Move to below her feet. Hold the foot up, supporting it under the calf or ankle, and press deeply on the sole with your thumb or the heel of the other hand, working round the contours of the foot. Finally, lower the foot to the floor and work on the toes. Work delicately on each toe, moving with small twiddlings of finger and thumb that feel all the tiny bones from the base to the tip. Then pull off at the tip, as if you were pulling off socks with toes in them. This feels lovely and liberating.

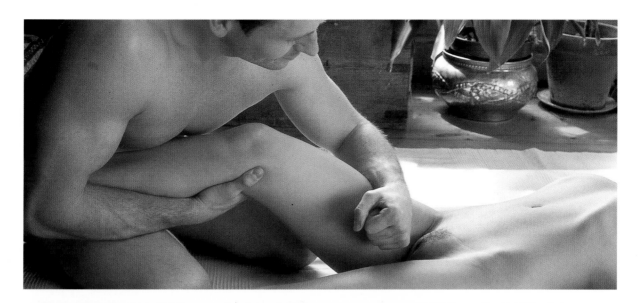

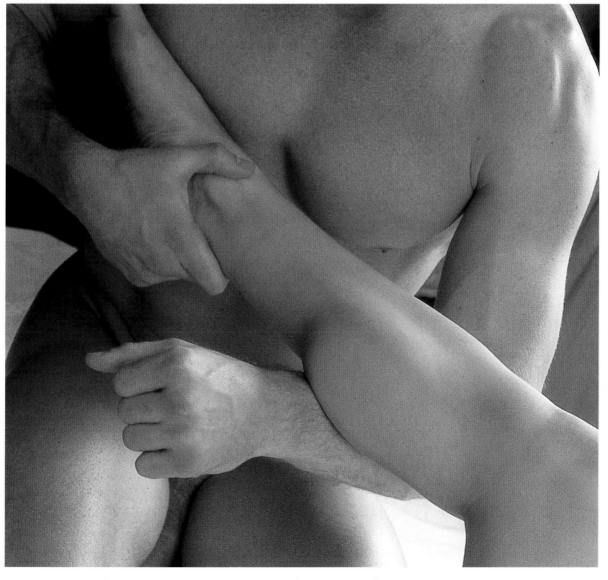

Belly and chest

Tension often locks the rib cage together tight like a corset. In massaging your partner's torso you will help her to free the ribs, breathe deeply and relax. Sit astride her upper legs facing her head. Place your palms lightly on her belly and ask her to breathe from here, so that her belly rises and falls beneath your hands. The shallow breaths we unconsciously take from the chest don't use the full capacity of the lungs, so stale air is never properly expelled and the blood doesn't get its maximum dose of oxygen. Really deep breaths can induce a pleasant feeling of lightheadedness.

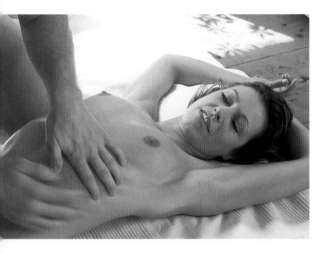

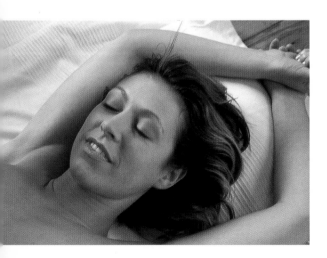

Sexual tension buster 5

1. With your partner lying on her back, start with broad gliding strokes over the whole torso. Don't forget that you are treating all body parts equally, so avoid the temptation to pay special attention to her breasts – in fact it's much more exciting for her that your hands will slide over and around them – it heightens anticipation for later.

2. Use two hands, palms down, to glide across the abdomen. Start with one under the breastbone and the other just above the pubic hair and move them in clockwise circles, with the lower hand brushing across the upper hand where they meet at the navel. Clockwise motion is important because it follows the movements of the bowel.

3. Next try a merry-go-round movement – while one palm describes a broad circle around the navel, the fingers of the other hand sketch a detailed spiral scribble along its path, giving a lovely lighthearted feeling.

4. Move to your partner's side to work the rib cage. Lean over to the opposite side of her body, cup your hands over her side and drag them alternately towards you, feeling with your fingers between her ribs and wriggling them loose. Apply firm pressure to avoid tickling. Work right down the side of the body, going over and over your tracks. Keep up these movements in a steady rhythm and it will feel to her as though lots of hands are touching her at once.

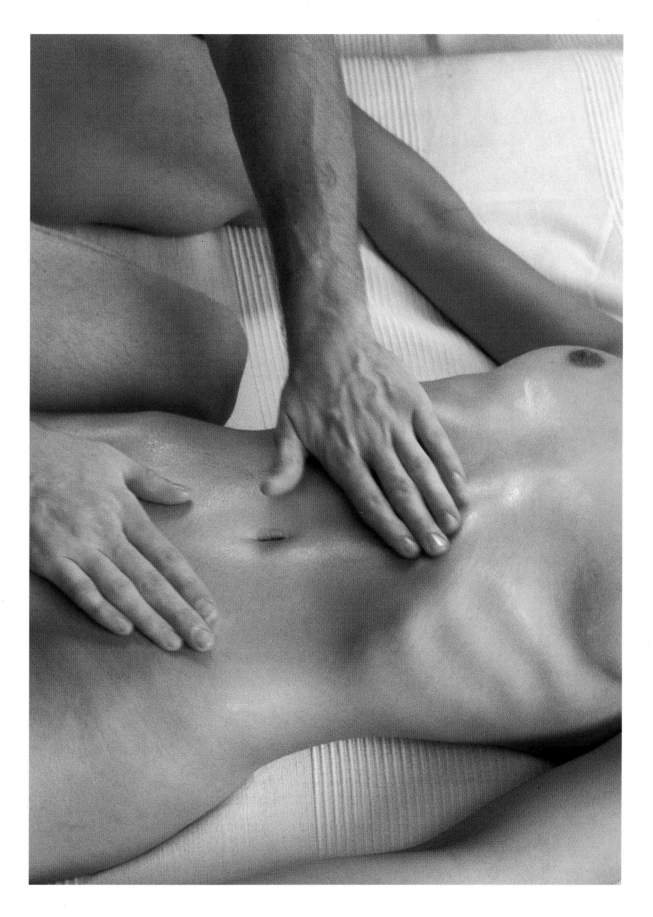

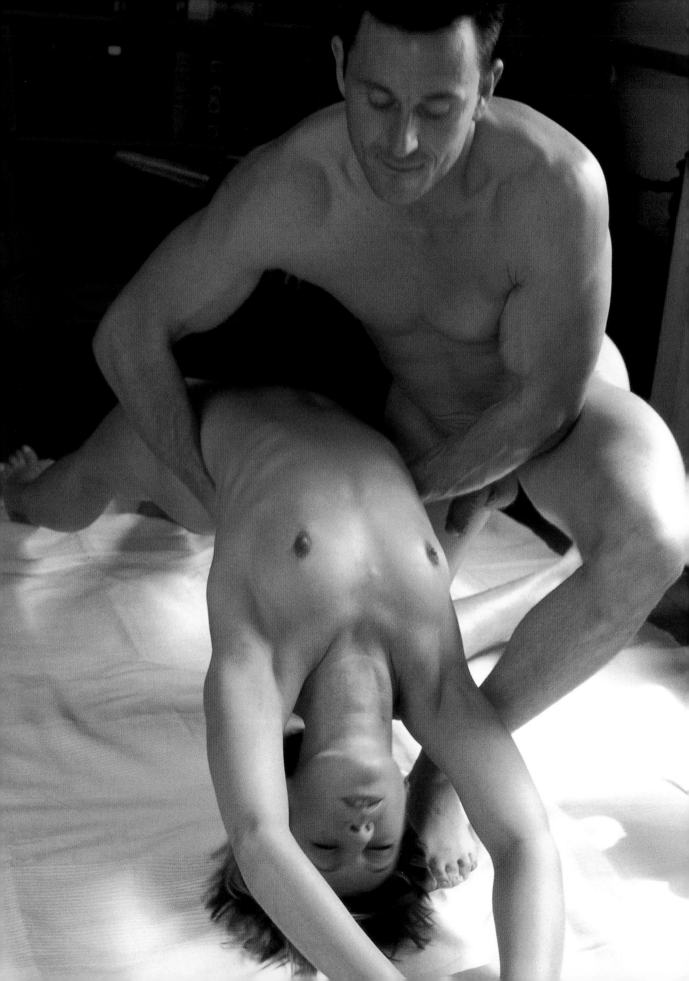

Lift and float

This is a movement that sends oxygenated blood flooding to the head to revive the brain – it's excellent for relieving headaches. To be picked up from a lying position and held is a powerfully emotive experience – it's quite possible that no one has done this for your partner since she was a baby, so it will fill her with feelings of love and of trust.

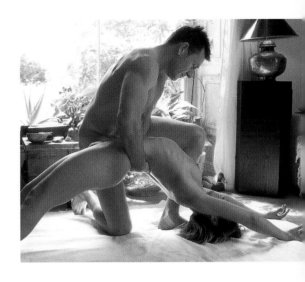

Take care

This is one of the few massage movements that requires strength – don't try to lift a partner who is much heavier than yourself. Watch out for your partner's neck as you lower her to the bed afterwards. Start with her neck at the edge of the bed so that her head slides naturally backwards as you lie her down.

Sexual tension buster 6

1. If your right leg is the stronger, kneel by your partner's left side; if your left leg is stronger, kneel by her right side. Clasp your hands with interlacing fingers beneath her waist. Tell her to keep her body completely relaxed and limp. Put your stronger foot forwards and raise yourself off the ground, lifting your partner's waist at your hips and bearing her weight on your leg.

2. Hold her in this position for 20 seconds or longer, then lower her down again, supporting her neck with one hand if you can.

3. Without losing contact, repeat the motion several times, so it feels to her as though a wave is carrying her to the shore. Even after the first lift, you should notice a difference. Her face will be slightly flushed, her eyes shining, and small tension lines will have disappeared.

And while you're there...

Finish with an all-over body stroke – a generous invigorating movement that joins her whole body from ankles to shoulders. Unless she is lying on a massage table and you can walk alongside her as your hands glide over her skin, you will have to change positions as you work. Try to do this without breaking contact or the flow of your stroke.

Start just above her ankles with one well-oiled palm and fingers cupping each leg. Push firmly and smoothly up the legs and over the torso with your fingertips touching. Let your hands part under her neck and move outwards over her shoulders.

Sweep your hands round her shoulders and back to her torso again just below the armpits. Run your hands right down her sides to the ankles again. Repeat several times to give a tingling, alive-all-over feeling.

Face and head

The sensual pleasures of rubbing cleansers and moisturizers into the skin every day and enjoying an occasional facial or relaxing scalp massage at the hairdresser's are treats that pass most men by. An erotic face and head massage is the answer. You won't need oil for this one.

Sexual tension buster 7

Let your intuition and your partner's responses guide you as you sit behind his head and try the following movements:

1. Starting with your fingers under his chin, sweep the flats of your hands up the sides of his face, pulling the flesh taut at the temples and following through with your fingers through his hair.

2. Work in tiny circles just below the jawbone, starting at the tip of the chin and moving right round to just under the ears.

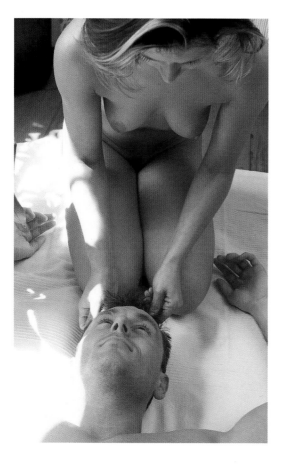

3. Join the tips of your index fingers under his nose and the tips of your middle fingers below his mouth. Pull your fingers towards the corners of his mouth, drawing a smile on his face around it. Let them follow under the cheekbones, up the sides of his face and over his ears.

4. Slide your fingers under the ears and work them firmly along the groove between the ear and the face. Wiggle and swirl the fingertips inside the ear flaps. Twiddle the earlobes between your fingers and thumb.

5. Working from the base of the neck, raise his head in both hands, stretch his neck, then rake with your fingertips through his hair as you let his head relax gently back on the pillow. At first he will probably keep his neck held stiff – tell him that you need to feel the weight of his head in your hands. This is a wonderful movement to relieve neck pain.

6. With your two index fingers, make small circling movements on the face at either side of the nostrils. Work up the sides of the nose then work the bridge, but avoiding the delicate skin around the eyes.

7. Cup the sides of the forehead in your hands and work with small circling movements from the bridge of the nose along the eyebrows, stretching them as you go. Very delicately smooth the skin under brows with outward sweeping fingertips.

8. Starting from the bridge of the nose, pass alternate hands lightly across the brow and into the hair.

9. Give the scalp an invigorating massage, whirling your thumbs and fingertips all over it. Finish by holding the top of his head in your hands.

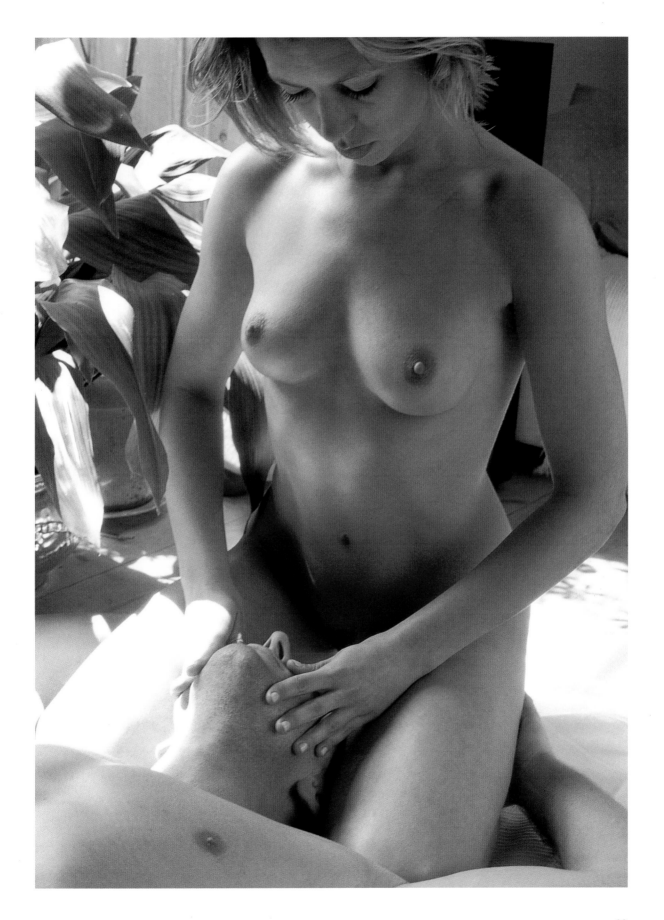

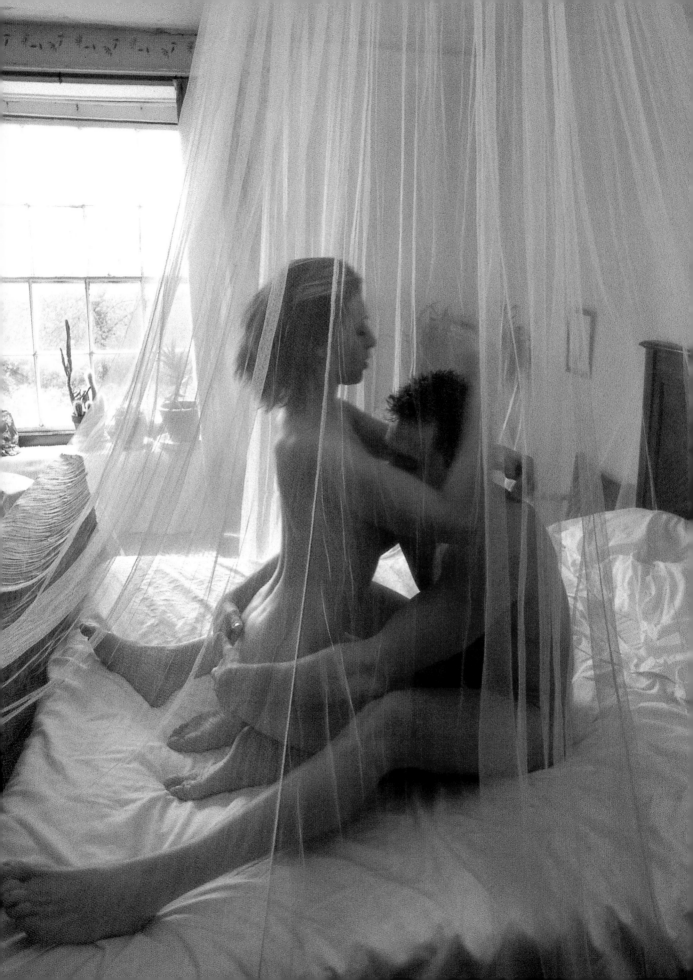

EXPLORE

To get the most fun out of sex you need to explore your own and your partner's responses in awesome detail and learn to play each other's body like a musical instrument. Study the sensitivity of your partner's main erogenous zones and, using different types of friction with tongue, fingers and genitals, discover the best way to arouse. Everyone has their own special lusts and needs. Then explore ways of varying the stimulation so you can speed up arousal or slow it down – control of timing is the secret of making sex last longer.

Kissing

Kissing is the greatest turn-on there is, because it shows your partner what an expert lover you are. To share a deep French kiss with full involvement of lips and tongues in a passionate clinch is the first sure sign in a new relationship that bed is on the agenda. New couples put all their erotic feelings into kissing – they kiss as if their whole lives depended on it – but sadly people who've been together a long time forget the joys and the urgency of intimate, imaginative mouth-to-mouth contact and may kiss only in bed before or during sex. Some stop kissing altogether – relationship counsellors know that the kiss is first to go when couples stop enjoying sex.

So what makes a great kisser?

Be imaginative with your lips and tongue. Use their mobility and suppleness to communicate your feelings.

Probe with your tongue seductively in your partner's mouth, but don't dart it in and out like a lizard or shove it aggressively down the throat – this won't be pleasant.

Try gently sucking on your partner's tongue or their lower lip.

Who takes the lead? Try alternating. Lead the kiss yourself or tune into your partner's kiss and follow their lead. Or play passive and let yourself be kissed – particularly good for a man who feels he's always expected to play the dominant role.

Pay attention to the corners of your partner's mouth with your tongue, pushing it inside the mouth to echo the feeling of the penis pushing inside the vagina.

Have your partner open their mouth and bare the tongue, then lick across it with generous broad strokes from corner to corner – an especially arousing kiss.

In a prolonged kissing session the shorter partner often gets a crick in the neck, so try kissing on the stairs or use a footstool.

What to do with your hands? Cradle your partner's face, support their neck, stroke their hair. Some people are driven wild by a finger gently inserted into their mouth along with your tongue.

Kiss other parts of the body, not just the mouth. Many women love having their palms, wrists, foreheads and eyelids gently kissed.

Finally, pay attention to oral hygiene! None of these delicious techniques will work if your breath is bad. Take yourself to the dentist and get your teeth sorted out. Give up smoking. Avoid alcohol and pungent foods – unless, of course, you're going to share it.

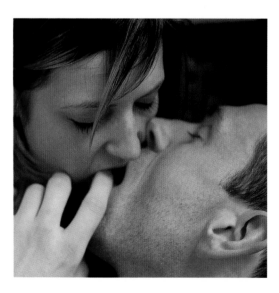

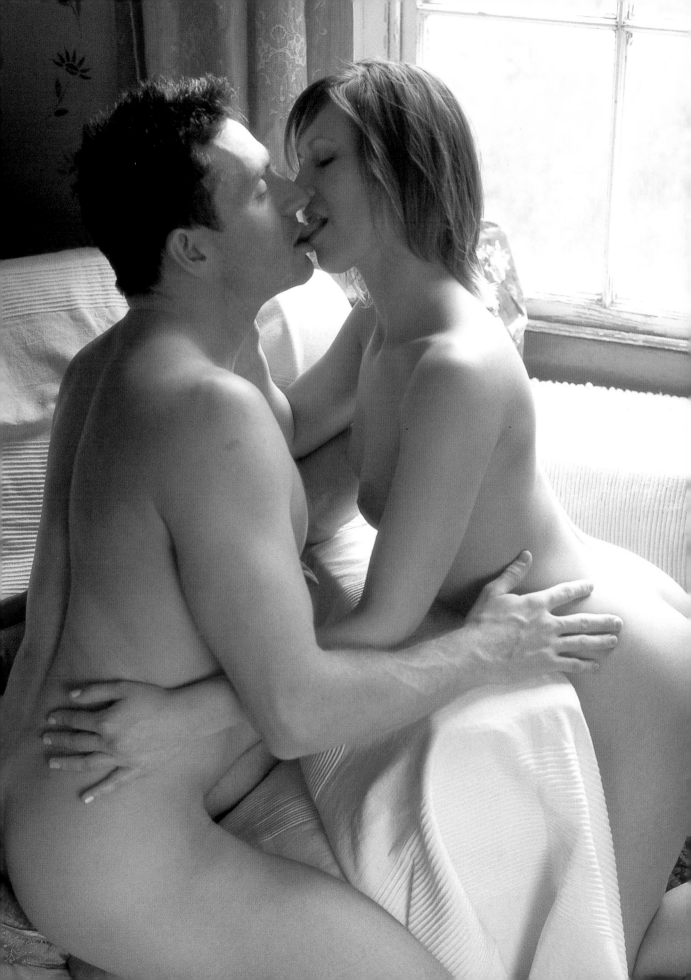

Secret erogenous zones

Did you know there's a theory that people with similar earlobes are unconsciously attracted to each other? How do yours match up? Never looked? And what other parts of your partner's body have you neglected to study? Giving your lover detailed attention is a powerful turn-on – you might be the first person to explore places like the crook of the arm, behind the knee or the nape of the neck since your lover was a small child. Which is why it will give him or her a tremendous feeling of being loved and wanted.

The ear

Some people just love having their earlobes nibbled and sucked. A few even adore to have their ears licked, with the tongue slowly swirling round the contours of the ear flap and flicking down inside. Ask first, in case your lover finds it ticklish or a turn-off.

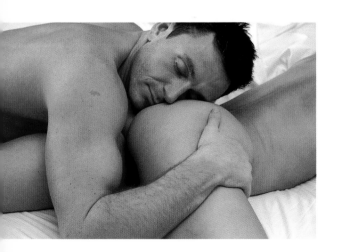

The feet

Try sucking your partner's toes one by one. Experiment with using the man's big toe as a penis substitute – some women find this very erotic. Short nails and smooth skin, please. It adds a new dimension to games of footsie under the table. And try a foot bath in scented hot water for tired feet – a lovely treat when one of you comes in exhausted from work.

The navel

Lick with the flat of your tongue in broad stokes, sweeping in a clockwise direction around the navel and circling inwards. Then hold your partner's buttocks with one hand, pressing the heel of the hand very firmly into the perineum and pulling upwards, and dance the tip of your tongue all around and over the belly button, exploring every tiny crevice. Hit the right nerve here and you'll send a tingling sensation streaking right down to the genitals.

The buttocks

There's lots of scope on this fleshy part for vigorous activity, such as kneading, playful smacks, sucking and nibbling – but don't neglect the sensitivity of the skin. Stroke the buttocks ever so lightly with your palm and fingertips, trailing your hand in lazy circles around their curves. Note that the buttocks make a wonderful pillow for relaxing after lovemaking.

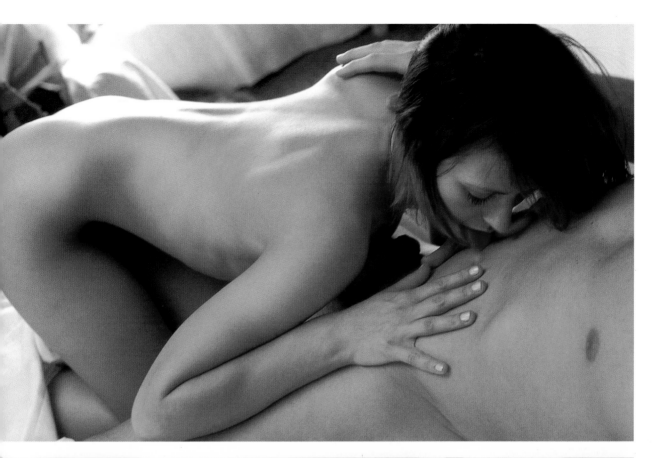

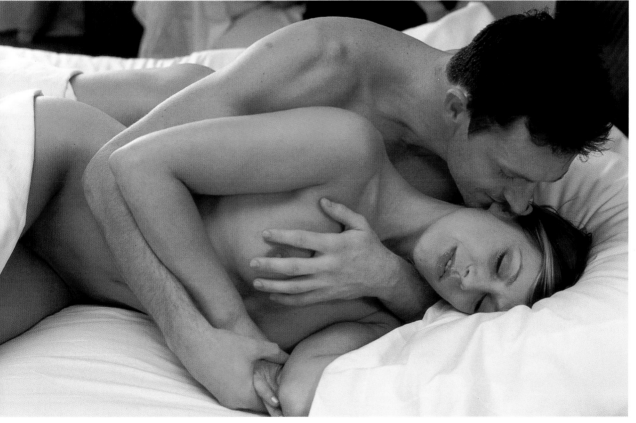

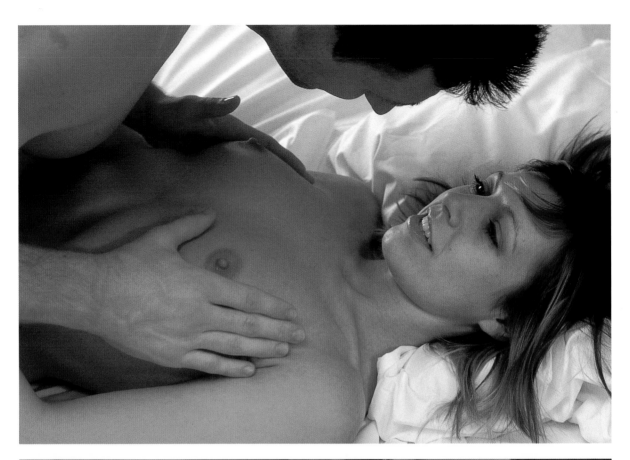

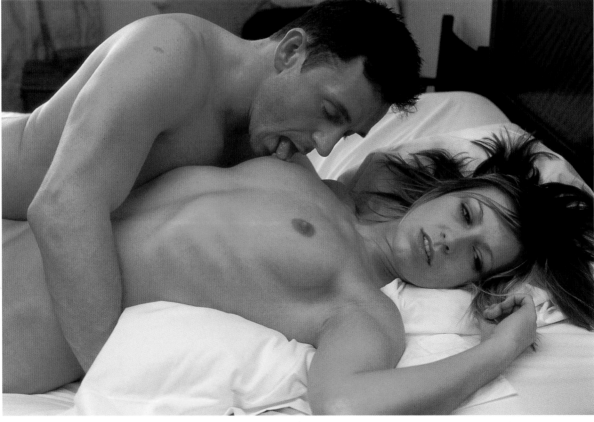

The breasts

Observe closely what happens to your partner's breasts during sex. All women react in different ways to arousal, but many develop a sexual flush that spreads from above the waist right across their chest. The areola – the dark disc around the nipple – may swell or get darker. In many women the nipples become erect. Some experience this during foreplay, and some more strongly or earlier in one breast than the other. Some women's breasts swell by as much as 25 per cent when they are aroused, and the veins in the breasts can stand out as blood flows into the area.

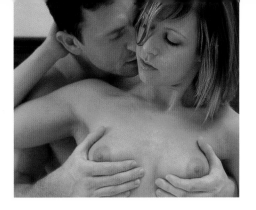

Sensitivity

The upper breast – from nine o'clock to three o'clock – is generally more sensitive than the lower breast. This discovery was made by scientists at Vienna University, who tested 150 women by blindfolding them and pricking their breasts with pins. Amazingly, they found that the nipple was the least sensitive part.

The Viennese scientists also discovered that large breasts are 24 per cent less sensitive than smaller breasts – because the nerve that transmits sensation from the nipple is stretched. Try gentle kneading and experimental nibbling.

Sagging breasts are least sensitive because nerves are stretched and compressed by the weight of the breasts. Consequently, she will feel better lying on her back. Push her breasts gently upwards as you fondle them.

Breast awareness

Be gentle and remember that breasts can be very tender around the time of a woman's period.

Cup and lift the breasts in both hands, massaging underneath them with a gentle circular motion.

Large areolas mean more nerve endings in this area, so don't stimulate nipples or areolas until she is fully aroused. Concentrate instead on caressing the outsides of the breasts.

Small areolas have fewer nerve endings and are less responsive. Work in tantalizing swirls with your tongue around the nipple, focusing on the areola and on the sensitive skin in the ten o'clock to two o'clock area of the breast.

Small breasts can be massaged in an all-over chest massage with the palms of the hands. Be firm as well as tender.

If she's had a successful breast implant, sensitivity shouldn't be impaired, but be careful how you move her breasts. Avoid vigorous handling and concentrate on feathery surface caresses with fingers or tongue.

Breastfeeding makes nipples extremely tender. Do your partner a favour and leave them for the baby. Lightly stroke swollen breasts on the less sensitive underside.

The vagina

Explore your partner's vagina as if you had never seen or felt a vagina before. Kneel on the floor with your partner lying with her bottom on the edge of the bed. Make yourself comfortable between her legs and begin by gently stroking the flats of your palms across her pubic hair and upper thighs. Gently part her legs and put her feet on your shoulders before you venture further.

Exploring the vagina

Stroke the whole area, just very lightly, then press your open lips to the skin of her upper thigh and breathe warm air on to it, circling the vulva and eventually homing in on it. Don't use your tongue. She will now be feeling warm, relaxed and very responsive. Part the pubic hair and very gently explore the shape of her vulva with your fingers. Delicately open the outer lips and this time breathe (not blow) warm air on to the open vulva without touching it with your lips.

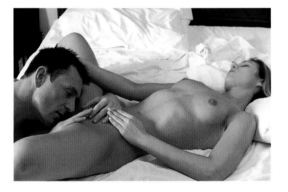

Inside the vulva

Begin to explore the vulva with your fingers, moving very slowly and lightly from the outside inwards. Don't touch her clitoris yet. Read her responses carefully and let them dictate your movement. Gradually build up rhythm and speed as if you were playing a living musical instrument. Use light flicking or rubbing movements, all the while using less pressure than you think she might be ready for so that her body movements continually beg you for more.

When you are sure the juices are flowing, dip your finger briefly into her vagina. Begin to explore it by darting in and out and let her thrust against you rather than press your fingers all the way in yourself. Keep withdrawing and playing the vulva with your fingertips.

Once you are deep inside her vagina, learn its shape, snugness and angle within her body. The better you know it, the more pleasure you can give her during intercourse, and the less chance you will have of hurting her by stabbing at the wrong angle. Right at the top of the vagina is something that feels a bit like the cap of a mushroom. This is the cervix, the neck of the womb.

Caution: Never blow into the vagina – it could cause serious harm.

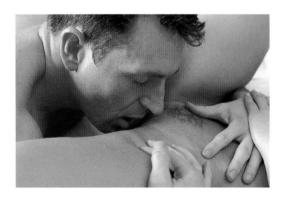

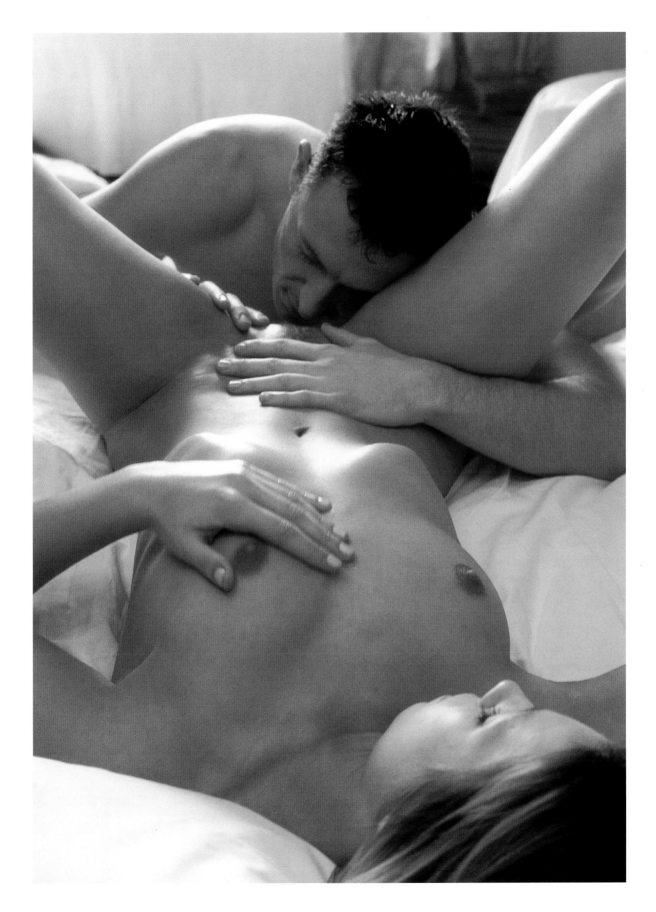

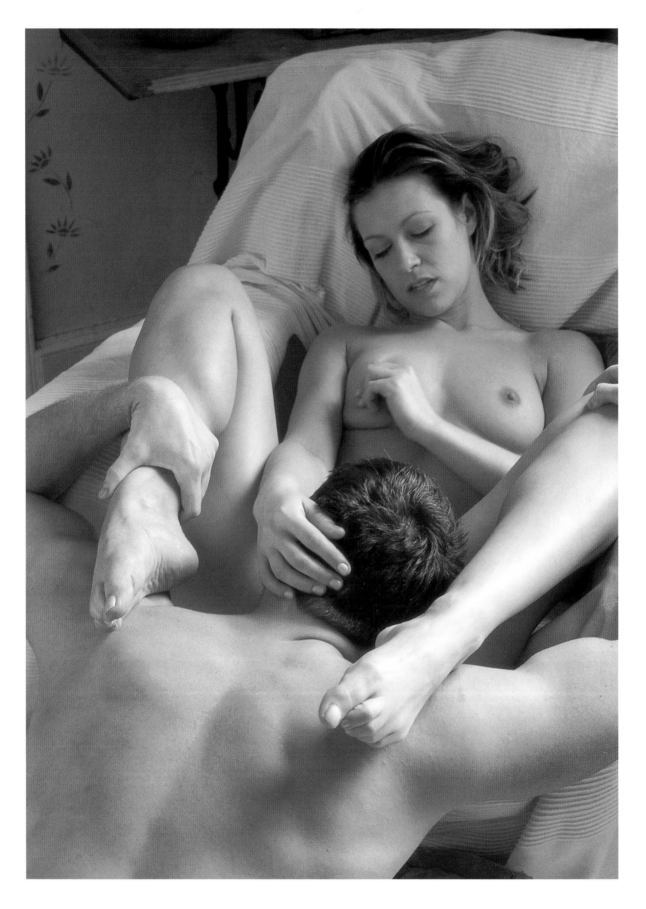

Cunnilingus

More women orgasm every time with oral sex than any other way because of the exquisite pleasure that the tongue can give with slippery, feathery or firm flicking movements over and around the clitoris. The sensitive tongue generally gives more powerful orgasms than the fingers, and the intimacy of the mouth to genital contact is also a powerful turn-on.

The most comfortable position

She lies on her back on the bed with her legs splayed and her knees up towards her stomach. You lie on your front with your head between her legs, supporting her thighs with your hands, which you can also use to brush her pubic hair out of the way and gently part her labia. Another good position is for her to lean back in a comfortable chair, with you sitting on the floor in front of her on a cushion.

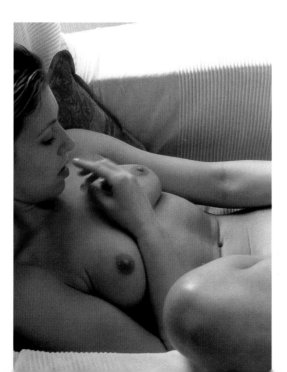

Licking tips

Every woman's vaginal juices taste different – salty, nutty or sweet. This is usually part of why you love her, but if you're worried about first-time hygiene, make bathing together part of your erotic menu.

Be very gentle and wait until she is fully aroused before making contact with the clitoris. The whole of the vulva will swell and flush, and the clitoris may well appear red and swollen from inside its hood.

A respondent in one survey said he plays what he calls 'the alphabet game' – writing capital letters with his tongue very slowly over his partner's open vulva, barely touching the clitoris as he passes it.

Get your partner to help you with what feels best. Rather than have her say: 'Up a bit, down a bit,' ask her to describe where she would like to be licked next by imagining her vulva as a clock face. Six o'clock, at the opening of the vagina, and twelve o'clock, right above the clitoris, are particularly sensitive areas.

Probe into her vagina with your tongue, then try gentle firm pressure all over the vulva, letting your tongue 'dance'. A repeated light rhythmic flicking across the clitoris will usually have the effect of inducing the tension that releases into orgasm.

Many women find the clitoris is too sensitive to touch after they come. Ask what she likes – often this is the best time for penetration.

Female orgasm

Male sexuality is pretty straightforward – men are usually quickly aroused and have no trouble reaching orgasm, in fact they often get there rather faster than they and their partners would like. But the female orgasm is more elusive – something of a mystery. In general, women have a slower and more complex sexual response and their orgasm depends on many factors, including how secure they feel as well as what their partner does to stimulate them.

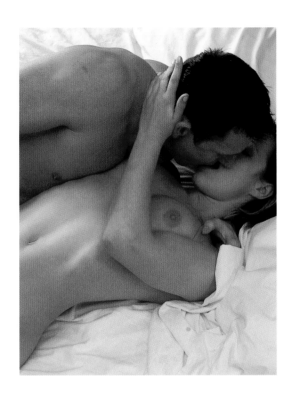

Inducing orgasm

Surveys show that penetration is the least likely way to induce orgasm in a woman. That's because in most positions the penis doesn't touch the clitoris – the little pea-shaped organ that hides under a hood of skin between the labia and above the entrance to the vagina. The clitoris is the epicentre of female pleasure, but that doesn't mean you should make a beeline for it – touch this highly sensitive organ only after plenty of foreplay has made both labia and clitoris swell with blood, much as the penis erects. This is the signal that she's truly ready for the climax.

Softly, softly

Before you even touch her genitals, arouse your partner with kisses – mouth to mouth and all over her body – and by cradling her in your arms and stroking her skin. The first genital contact can be a light brushing of the hand across the pubic hair. Read her response and when she is ready, explore with your fingers inside her vulva.

The best way to give a woman an orgasm is with oral sex (cunnilingus). Spend as much time on it as it takes before you penetrate her and have your own first orgasm. Once she knows you are prepared to lavish unlimited attention on her she will relax and be able to lose herself in the sheer bliss of what she is feeling – and there's nothing more likely to boost a man's ego than making his partner come in this way.

Try a session where she undresses completely but you stay dressed (wearing something non-constricting like tracksuit bottoms) until you have given her an orgasm.

Many women confound the 'complex response' theory by being able to make themselves come really quickly – as fast as men can – when they masturbate or use a vibrator. This is down to a combination of being in the right mood and knowing exactly which parts of themselves to touch and how. Ask your partner to show you what she does – then try to do it yourself under her guidance.

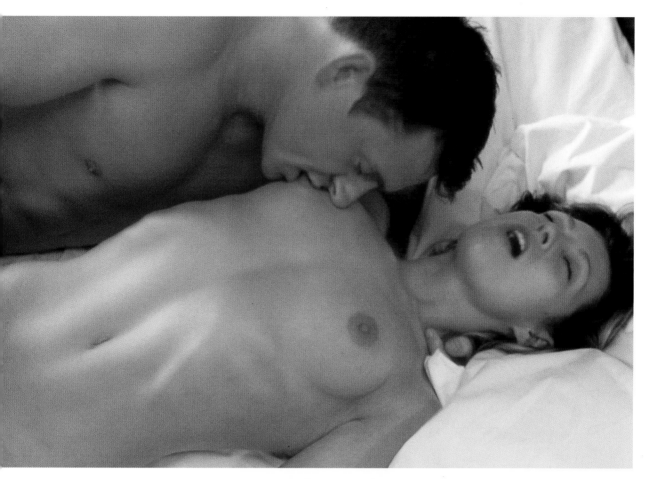

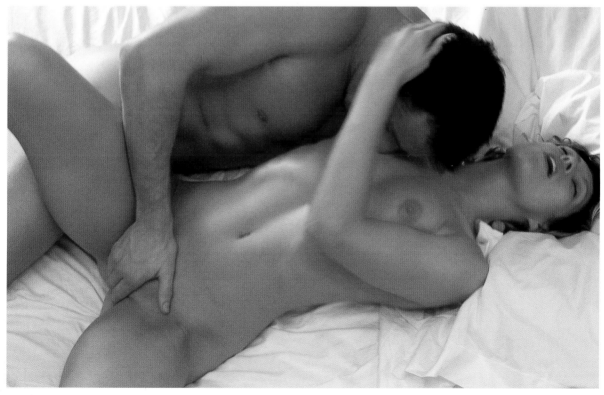

The G-spot

Controversy surrounds the mysterious G-spot — a sensitive area half way up the front wall of the vagina. It was named after its discoverer, Ernst Grafenberg, who claimed that when it was stimulated, a woman would have an orgasm accompanied by an ejaculation of sexual fluid very similar in chemical composition to the secretions of the male prostate gland.

Does the G-spot really exist?

In one US survey, 40 per cent of women claim to ejaculate in this way, but another survey shows fewer than 5 per cent believe that it has happened to them. Conduct your own experiments with your fingers or concentrate on sex positions that target the spot.

If so, where?

Grafenberg, working in the 1940s, advised that the newly discovered erotic hot spot swelled when stimulated with firm, deep, continuous pressure, becoming a tiny female erection. The best way to do this is for the woman to lie on the bed on her front, legs slightly apart and buttocks slightly raised. Insert two fingers into her vagina, palm down, and explore the front wall of the vagina. Ask her to tell you what feels good. She may have a brief sensation that she's about to

urinate, which gives way to erotic pleasure. If there is any ejaculate, take a good look at it. Some say it's colourless, some say it's milky like semen. Others believe that due to loss of pelvic muscle control, some women squirt urine as they come.

Ancient wisdom

The idea that women ejaculate goes back to the ancient Greeks and beyond. Here's what Hippocrates wrote in 400BC: 'During intercourse, when a woman's genitals are vigorously rubbed and her womb titillated, lustfulness overwhelms her down below, and the feeling of pleasure and warmth pools out through the rest of her body. A woman's body also produces an ejaculation, which happens at the same time inside the womb, which has become drenched with wetness, as well as on the outside, because the vagina is now gaping and open.'

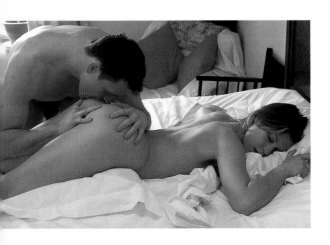

Trying it out

Experiment with stimulating the G-spot during intercourse. Try it with the woman lying on her front and the man entering from behind, or the woman lying on her back with a bolster cushion under her buttocks, or on all-fours, doggy style. If the man lies down and she sits astride facing his feet, she can control the angle of penetration herself. If you prove the existence of the G-spot, great — if you prove it doesn't exist, you will at least have had fun trying.

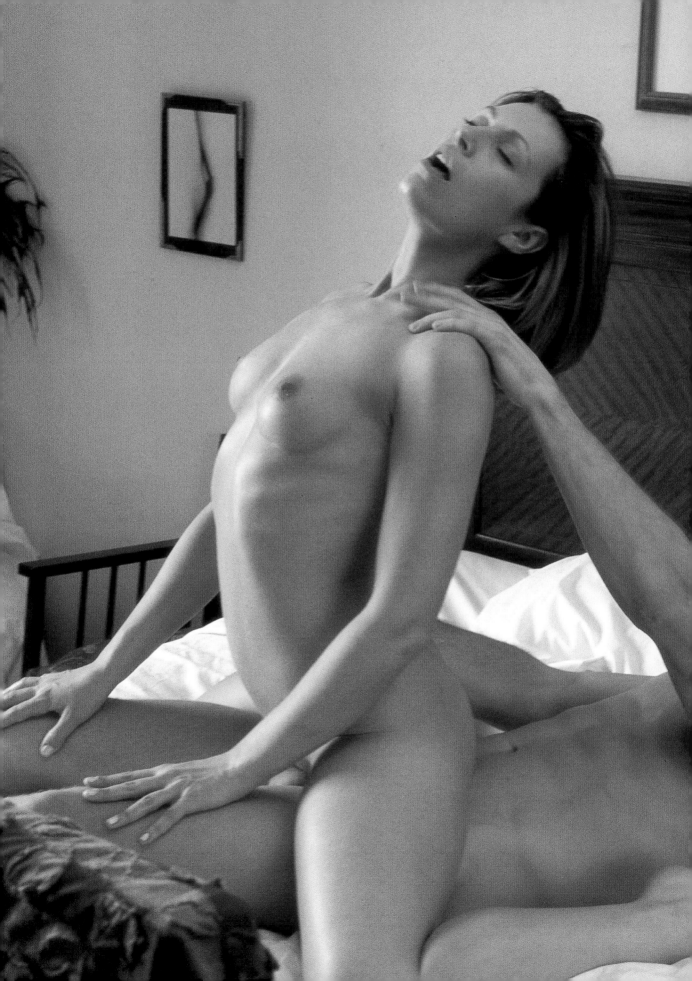

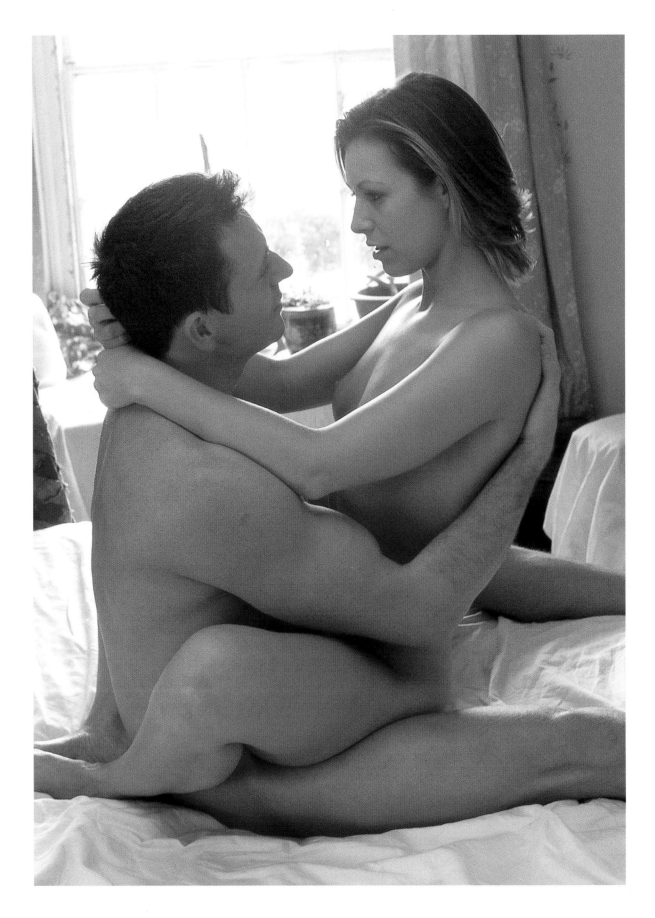

The pelvic floor muscles

The pelvic floor is a network of muscle that supports the organs of the pelvis – the bladder, genitals and anus. You can feel where it is by contracting the muscles at the front that would stop a flow of urine, and those at the back that would stop a bowel movement. Toning these very same muscles – the pubococcygeus, or PC for short – will give both sexes a more intense and controlled orgasm.

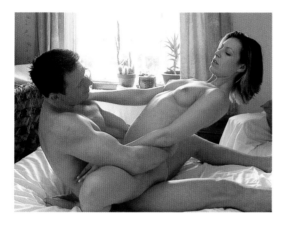

The female PC

In women, the muscles of the pelvic floor are often seriously weakened by childbirth, particularly if labour has been long and difficult. The result is that the vagina loses its snug and responsive elasticity and feels slack and loose during lovemaking, which can be disappointing for both partners. Sometimes there are problems with bladder control – especially while laughing or coughing, and in severe cases, damaged pelvic floor muscles can lead to a prolapse of the womb.

PC exercises

Keep your PC muscles supple with Kegel exercises (so called after their inventor) by repeatedly contracting them as strongly as you can for 10 seconds, then relaxing them. Men, and women who have not recently given birth, should aim at 150 contractions a day. The advantage with these exercises is that you can do them anywhere, at any time, without anyone knowing – in the bath, in the office, on the bus...

Exercise tips

After childbirth, a woman should exercise twice a day for 20 minutes to help the muscles recover and prevent further weakening.

Vary the exercise: start with the front, bladder-connected muscles, then move on to the back, anus-connected muscles. Or alternate between the two.

For the scientifically minded, a machine called a perineometer has been invented by an American gynaecologist. A tube with a rubber bulb at the end of it is connected to a box with a dial. The woman puts the bulb inside her vagina and squeezes – the strength of the contraction is registered on the dial.

Men will develop a stronger and more sensitive erection by 'waving the wand'. Sit on the edge of the bed. Locate the muscles that move your penis up and down and from side to side, and flex them for about 10 minutes every day.

Finally, share the fun while monitoring each other's progress. Flex your muscles while making love. As soon as one of you starts this game, you should both keep absolutely still, communicating only with these muscles. This is a delicious way to have an orgasm.

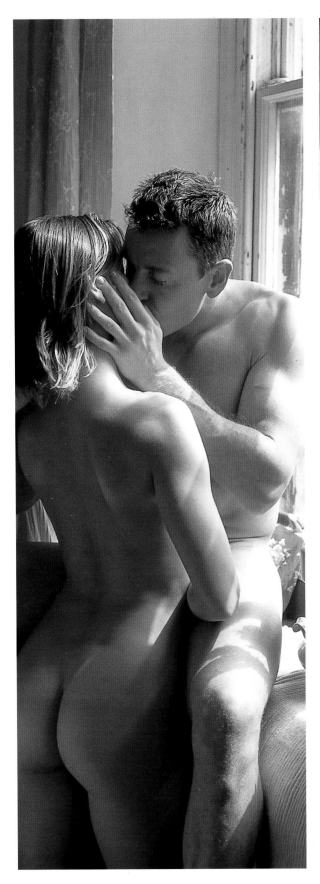
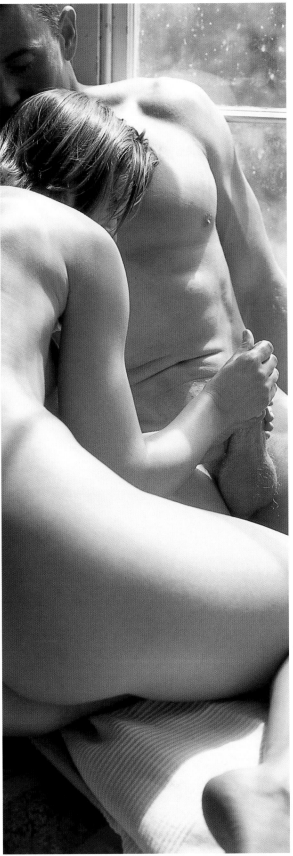

Male masturbation

You can learn a lot about how to handle your partner's penis by watching him masturbate. And then you can improve on his repertoire by adding imaginative variations of your own.

Handling tips

It can be daunting for a man to have his partner 'try' to give him an erection by direct manipulation – pressure to perform is never a turn-on. So wait, and don't handle his penis until it's erect and actually aching to be touched.

Be confident, firm and leisurely in your movements. Give him the feeling that you're totally in control – and in no hurry.

If he is circumcised, concentrate on the shaft, moving the penile skin up towards the glans and then back down again.

While you are masturbating him, tune into his needs. Tantalize him by changing rhythm or speed and by varying the angle and pressure.

Try drumming your fingers on the shaft as if you were playing the flute.

Is he circumcised or not?

Circumcision is often carried out on male babies for reasons of religion or tradition. It is the surgical removal of the foreskin, so a circumcised adult penis lacks the hood of skin that covers the glans (tip) of a flaccid uncircumcised penis. Surveys suggest that women prefer the neater look of circumcised men, but find it easier to masturbate an uncircumcised penis.

In the US there is a movement among circumcised men to 'regrow' their foreskins by exercising and with weights. Some men say that the unsheathed glans loses its sensitivity as it rubs against clothing, robbing them of the more exquisite sexual sensations.

The technique

1. Brush the flat of your palm along the insides of his legs, over his balls and quickly and lightly up the shaft, hardly touching the tip. Do this several times, increasing the pressure. His penis will strain up to meet your hand.

2. 'Weigh' his penis in your hand. Lift it up and let it drop back – smack – on to his belly. Watch it bounce. Repeat.

3. Hold the shaft firmly in your hand and squeeze repeatedly, first very gently and then more firmly, as you passionately kiss his mouth.

4. Walk your fingers in mischievous steps up the shaft and very lightly tickle the tip as it rises to meet you.

5. If he is uncircumcised, hold the penis in your hand and make a snugly fitting circle with your forefinger and thumb just below the glans. Slowly pull down the foreskin. Stop. Squeeze. Raise the foreskin again. Take your time. Gradually build up a rhythm.

6. Towards the end, keep up the pressure and speed coolly and with control – he needs no distractions now – and when you feel his body tense for orgasm hold on and carry through, not stopping until he subsides.

The testicles

Literally 'witnesses' to the sex act (as in 'testify'), the testicles are the glands where sperm and male hormones are produced. They hang outside the body in the scrotal sac for a reason – sperm need a cooler-than-body temperature to survive. Which is why tight pants and hot baths are not good for conception. In sex play, the testicles are often neglected. Perhaps this is because everyone knows they are extremely pain-sensitive – but they also respond well to gentle or firm stimulation and many men adore having them caressed and licked.

Handling the testicles

1. First, take a good look. One may hang slightly lower than the other, and one is most probably bigger. When you cup them in your hand, note their shape and weight. They swell slightly with arousal, and move mysteriously under the scrotal skin, creating an effect like waves out at sea. Just before ejaculation, they tighten and rise up under the penis, ready to testify to what is happening.

2. Pay attention to his inner thighs – he may be surprised at how sensitive they are. Stroke them fleetingly with the palms of your hands, then push them apart and breathe hot air on them, barely touching them with your lips. Nuzzle up to his balls and, with your tongue, trace the 'seam' between them, pushing them up like a seal doing tricks. Then playfully lick first one then the other from below, working round the sides to the top.

3. Pay attention to the perineum – that's the place in between the scrotum and the anus – massage it with little walking steps with your fingers, pressing quite firmly, then swoop into feathery strokes all over the balls, alternating with cupping them in your hand and 'testing their weight'.

4. With a firm tongue, lick vigorously and repeatedly from the upper corner of his thigh towards the point where penis and scrotum join. Then concentrate on licking the testicle nearest to you with the same firm motion, occasionally 'accidentally' straying on to the root of the erect penis, which you are pretending to ignore.

5. After licking his testicles all over with little flicking licks, probing between them with the tip of your tongue to define their shape, nibble them with your lips, lick salaciously with the flat of your tongue, and gradually take one or both balls in your mouth. Use your lips and tongue only to manoeuvre them - make sure you keep your teeth covered by your lips.

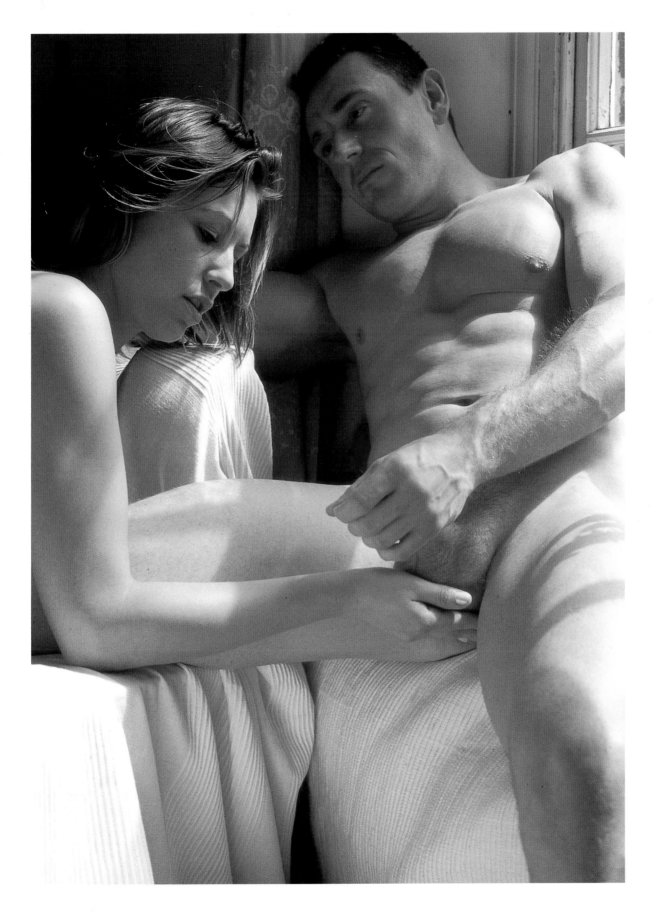

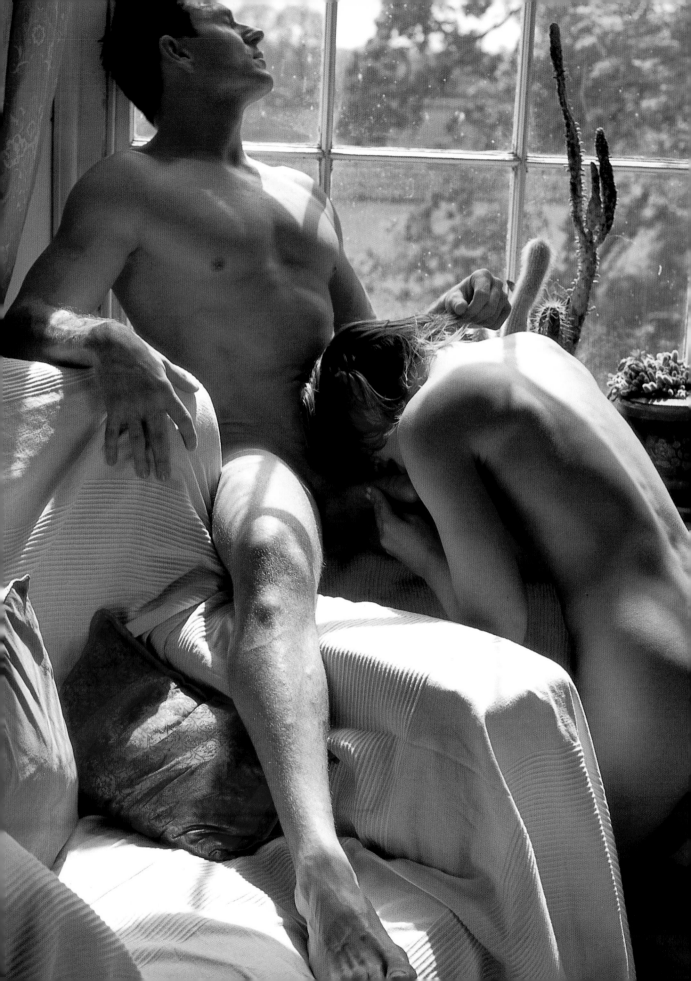

Fellatio

Cleopatra was honoured with the title 'the great swallower'. Her enemies spread envious rumours of her fellating dozens of soldiers in her army in one night. If you haven't swallowed it before, masturbate or fellate your partner to orgasm and dip your finger in the semen as it squirts out of his urethra. It feels warm and may taste nutty, salty or sweet, depending on what he has been eating and drinking. If he isn't well, it may taste bitter. If you like the taste, the best time to swallow it is immediately on ejaculation, as it becomes cloudy and more viscous as it cools.

Lick and suck

During fellatio, the woman, not the man, should be in control. How deeply she takes him into her mouth is down to her. In any case, some penises are too big for this and some mouths too small. There are plenty of more enjoyable and sophisticated ways to give fellatio than simply thrusting in the mouth. Use your imagination...

The technique

Be prepared to move around your partner's body as you lick and suck his penis, so you can enjoy it from every angle.

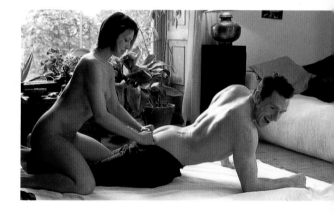

1. Nuzzle the shaft with the inside of your lips and apply pressure with the flat of your tongue as your mouth moves up and down towards the tip. Start at one side, move up and down the penis on top of him, then continue with the other side. Be energetic and thorough.

2. Hold the penis in your hand and, lubricating it with plenty of saliva and/or almond oil, masturbate it slowly, lavishly licking and tickling the tip with your tongue. Keep up well-lubricated flowing movements, alternating all the time between hands and tongue, so he hardly knows where the sensation is coming from. Let your mouth follow your hand in a smooth rhythm.

3. Now suck the tip of the penis with greedy sucking noises and lots of saliva, moving your hand rapidly and lightly up and down the shaft, and tickling the opening of the urethra with the tip of your tongue.

4. Feel his whole body tense, then spasm as he comes. Some men need you to carry on licking and sucking through several spasms, but with others, the glans becomes so sensitive that they can't bear contact any longer.

5. If you are not going to swallow the ejaculate, try letting it squirt on to your lips and fingers and massaging it into the still throbbing penis until ejaculation stops and it subsides.

Making it last

Great sex is all about timing. And some of the difficulty in getting the timing right lies in the fact that women have a slower and more complex sexual response than men – so it's all about the man keeping cool and slowing down while the woman heats up. Since the quickest way for a man to come is to get straight on with it and thrust powerfully and rhythmically until he ejaculates, it follows that to make sex last longer, get more out of it and give your partner a better time, you should not rush things. So concentrate on pleasing your lover.

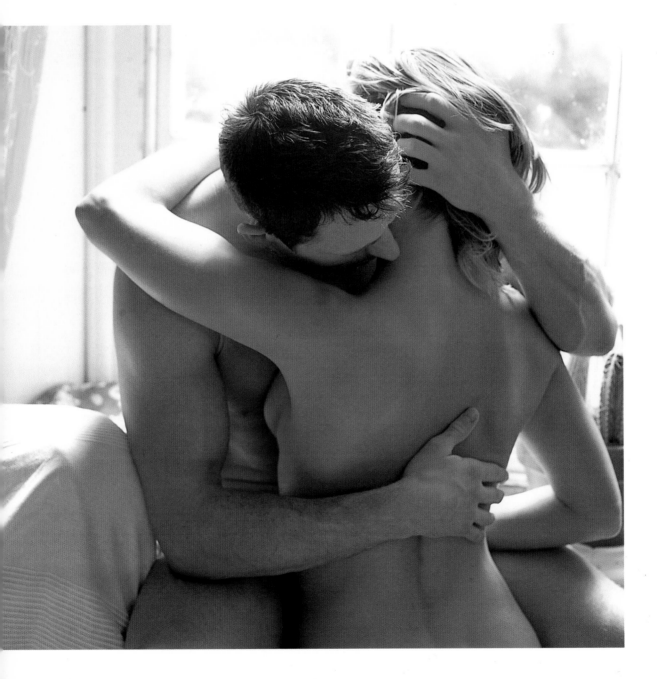

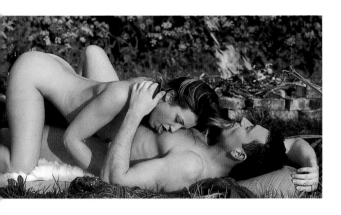

Pacing yourselves

Spend lots of time on foreplay, give her an orgasm first with your fingers or tongue, then move on to intercourse, but keep varying the position – sometimes with you on top, sometimes she will want to be on top, and you may also want to break off to give or receive oral sex.

Variety is the key – make a change every time you feel yourself about to lose control. And don't be shy about taking a break altogether – you're not in some kind of athletics championship. Stop and relax. Have a drink, or cuddle and talk. Your partner will cool down sexually much more slowly than you, so she'll be very responsive when you want to begin again.

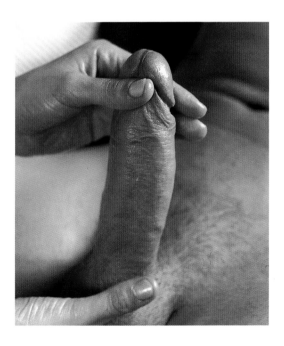

More tips for lasting longer

Try Kegel exercises (also called pelvic floor exercises, see page 47) to give you greater muscular control as well as more intense orgasms.

As you get nearer to orgasm, the testicles rise up tightly under the penis. To slow you down, stop thrusting, stay still, and gently hold your testicles down using the palm of one hand – or get your partner to do this for you. Wait a while before you begin again.

The stop-start technique involves just that – every time you reach a peak of excitement and feel yourself about to let go, stop, and without withdrawing, stay very still inside her until you feel the urgency has passed and you can begin to move again.

Your partner will enjoy helping you with the squeeze technique. Get her to masturbate you with her thumb on the frenulum – the skin on the underside of the penis just below the head, and her fingers just under the coronal ridge. When you feel you're about to come, she stops and squeezes for a couple of seconds, then releases. The squeeze will make you partly lose your erection, and once you have subsided a bit, she can start again. Do this until you can't stand it any more – then you will have a powerful orgasm.

Coming together

Some couples claim that simultaneous orgasm is the best thing that ever happened to them, while others find it a bit bewildering – the pleasure of your partner's orgasm is lost behind the explosion of your own, leaving you wondering what happened. You're not missing anything if it doesn't happen to you, but you can have a lot of fun experimenting with timing. It will add to your knowledge of each other's sexual responses and help make sex last longer. Since most couples find that the man usually gets orgasmic before the woman, here are a few tips to slow him down and speed her up.

Slowing a man down

Use lots of lubricant to create less friction, because friction is what stimulates you.

Avoid building up a thundering rhythm. Vary your thrusts between slow and deep and quick and shallow, but avoid pulling out so much that you stimulate the head of the penis as you drive back in again. Then combine the two – try going in slow, low and deep and coming out fast, pulling your body upwards as you do so. With you on top this stimulates the sensitive front of the vagina.

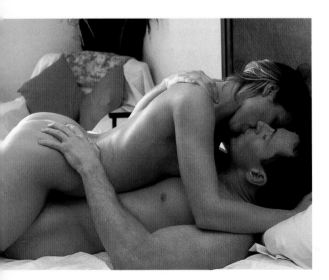

If you're getting too excited, withdraw and give her oral sex. Don't worry about going limp for a while, her increased arousal will soon get you going again. Before you go back to base give her a long erotic kiss on the mouth – many women are highly aroused by the mixture of love juices.

Speeding a woman up

Woman on top is always good as it gives her the opportunity to set the pace. She faces your toes to feel the pressure of the penis on the front wall of the vagina and get deep penetration.

Try another woman on top position: she faces your head and lies on your chest. She needs to be very vigorous as she drags her body upwards. She clenches the vaginal muscles and really tugs at your penis as if she were using her hand. She grinds back down in a circular motion, then drags up again – exquisite for both of you.

She sits on your lap facing away from you. While she rocks tightly back and forwards, you hold her labia open with one hand and fondle around her clitoris with the fingers of the other, giving her a stretched-to-bursting feeling that she wouldn't get if you actually touched her clitoris.

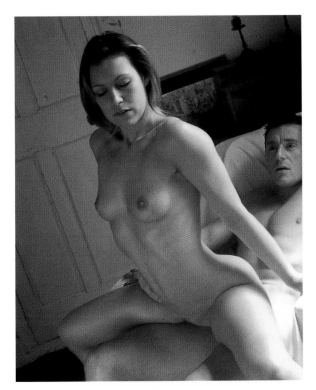

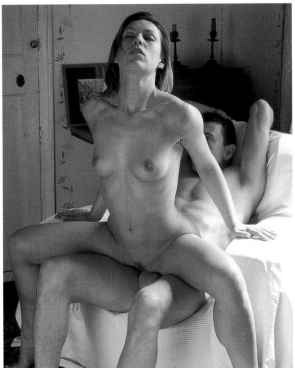

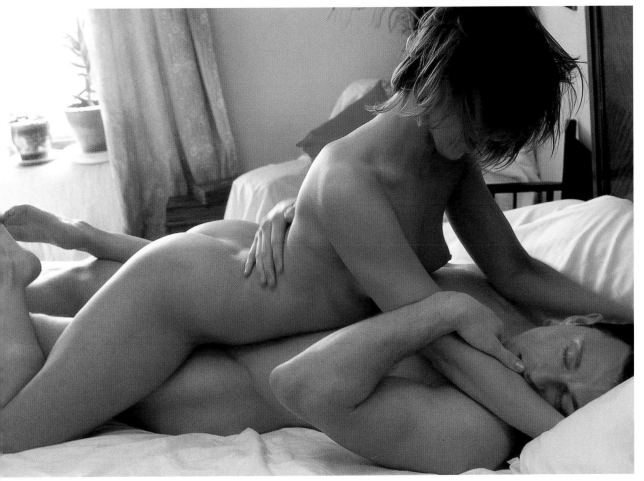

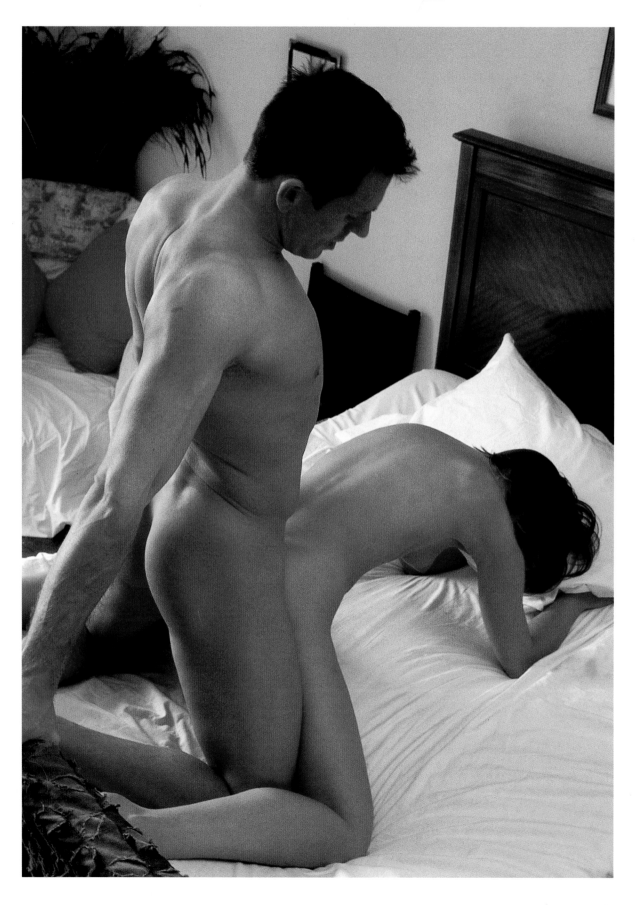

Anal sex

Anal sex among heterosexual couples has been practised throughout history for pleasure, to avoid breaking a girl's hymen and taking her virginity, or to avoid the risk of pregnancy or the messiness of menstrual blood. However, there are taboos against anal sex in many societies, and in some parts of the world – not least in several states of America – the practice is illegal: a man can be imprisoned for having anal sex even within marriage.

Trying it out

For some people the idea of anal sex is a complete turn-off, but if you want to try it, make sure your partner is fully aroused and completely relaxed before you begin. She should be pushing out with the anal muscles rather than holding them tight, or it could hurt.

Lubricate well with a water-based lubricant and proceed gently, at first just entering the anus with the tip of the penis and resting there a while, then working with and not against the muscles of the anus as they gradually allow you in. Let her dictate how deeply and strongly you thrust.

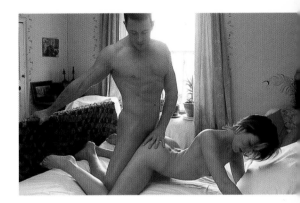

Tricks to try

Gently finger your partner's anus while you give him or her oral sex or during intercourse. Some like a finger to slide in and out of the anus.

For a woman, anal penetration feels quite different to vaginal sex. The anal sphincter clenches tightly on to the penis. Deep anal penetration can be the best way to stimulate the G-spot at the front wall of the vagina. Her partner can simultaneously insert a finger into the vagina, or one of them can manually stimulate her clitoris.

The male prostate gland can be stimulated during anal penetration. It is located about 5 cm (2 inches) inside the rectal passage towards the front of the body. Firm pressure applied here can lead to orgasm.

Caution

The lining of the rectum is thinner and more easily damaged than the vaginal wall, which means that anal sex is an effective way of an infected person transmitting the HIV virus that causes AIDS. Fingernails could also easily snag the membrane and transmit infection. So be scrupulous with hygiene and always use a condom or a latex glove.

Don't penetrate the vagina after the anus without washing thoroughly, or you could transfer bacteria from one to the other. Also take great care if inserting a sex toy into the anus – the rectal passage is capable of sucking objects up inside itself. So make sure your dildo is flared at the bottom so it won't disappear, as well as having no rough edges.

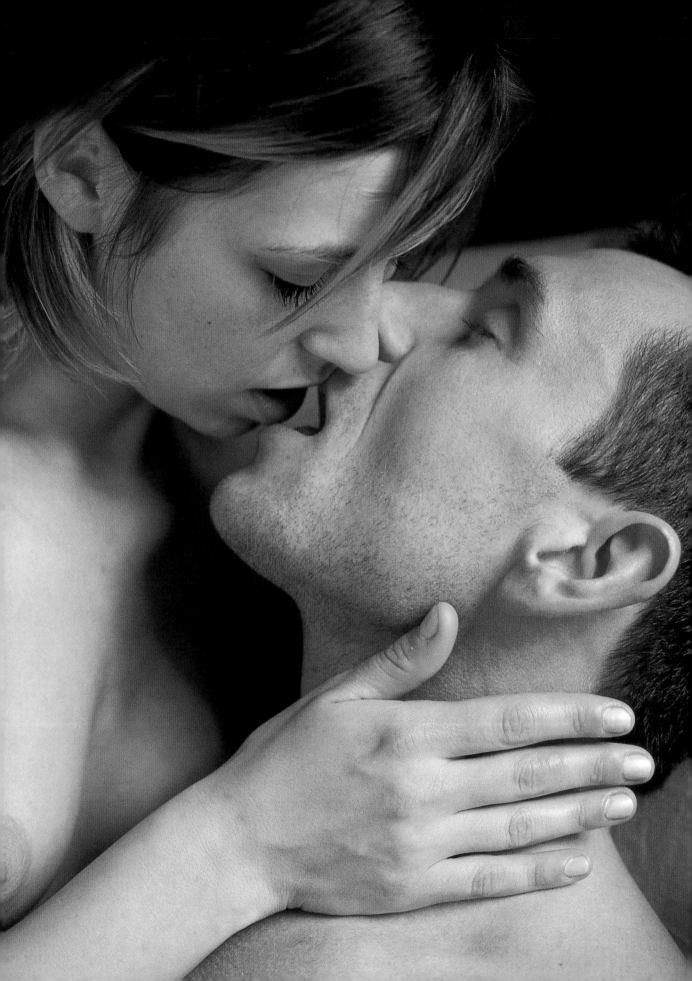

DISCOVER...

...new sensations – the power of
perfume to relax, stimulate and
reawaken erotic memories, the
novelty of a massage with the
tongue, nipples or hair. Play a sexy
guessing game and develop your
lover's sensitivity to touch with a
blindfold. Add the excitement
of making love in unexpected
locations – get swept away by
spontaneity and enjoy sex you'll
never forget. Learn new techniques
to improve your sexual expertise
and your lover's responsiveness,
and add spice to your love life by
acting out your fantasies. Discover
the secret of keeping your sex life
alive with imagination and variety.

How to build up to sex

A woman can make love passionately but she won't give all of herself sexually unless she feels totally secure. A really aware man who wants to give his partner an emotionally safe place in which to let go and express her sexuality without inhibitions will understand that, for a woman, sex begins way before you get to the bedroom. It lies in the way you speak to her, look at her and touch her all the time. That doesn't mean that your manner should be sexually loaded, but it should express your affection and your love.

That loving feeling

Feeling really loved is the best aphrodisiac a woman can have. So ask her about herself and don't forget to listen while she tells you! Touch her a lot – give her a hug, stroke her back, kiss the top of her head. Pay her small attentions to show that you think of her when you aren't together – phone to ask how she is, buy her flowers and bizarre little presents that don't cost much but will touch her heart.

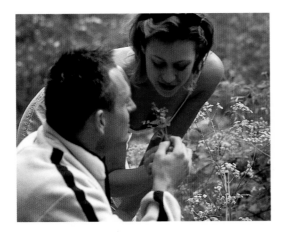

Seven ways to boost your partner's libido

Tell her you really love her and care about her deeply. There's nothing a woman likes to hear more than this. Men often take the fact that they love their partners for granted, and when asked if this is still the case, say something sarcastic like: 'Well, I wouldn't still be with you if I didn't, would I?' Your partner will take this as a put-down, and if she's feeling slightly insecure it will make her more anxious still. So tell her you love her when she's not even expecting it – it will do wonders for her ego.

Talk about your commitment and make plans together. To affirm that your relationship stretches out towards a positive future is a real morale booster.

Take her somewhere special on your own. It needn't be expensive – a long walk together can be just as memorable as a meal out.

Offer to give her a massage. See pages 10-29 for ideas.

Make her a delicious meal at home with wine, candlelight and chocolates. Book the evening in advance, but do all the planning and preparation yourself. Keep the menu a surprise. Don't let her help out.

Put little notes where she will see them – under her pillow or in the book she's reading. Send her postcards – even if you live together.

Do all these things often.

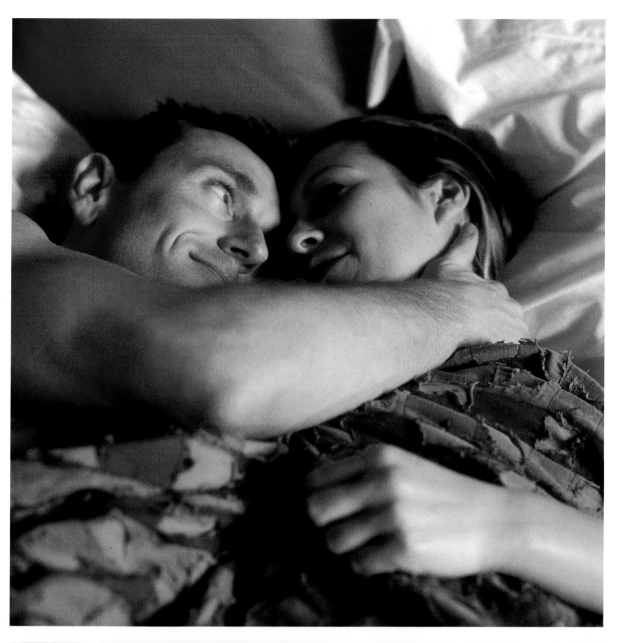

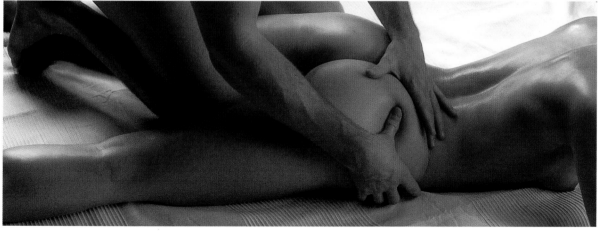

Lubrication

Sex is all about movement – rubbing, sliding, slipping, pushing, licking, stroking – and none of these movements can happen without lubrication. Some women's vaginas are awash with sexual secretions, while others are much drier. Dryness is also a natural accompaniment to the menopause. It doesn't have to mean you don't want sex, but it does make sex less comfortable unless you use a lubricant.

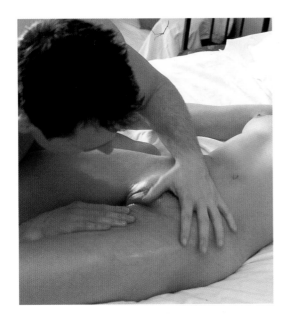

Almond oil

Almond oil is an excellent choice of lubricant. It is often used as a base for aromatherapy oils, so it has much more pleasant connotations than tubes of lube, which look medicinal. Decant it into a pretty bottle if you like (it usually comes in brown glass).

The main advantage of almond oil is that it has only a faint, sweet nutty taste, which does not spoil the flavour of human skin or juices. This makes it great for oral sex. It is also colourless, non-sticky, and delightful to use.

Introduce almond oil as part of an erotic massage, then zoom in on the genitals – his as well as hers. Used as a prelude to every sex encounter, erotic lubrication will become an ardent part of lovemaking and one that often allows a woman to have an early climax.

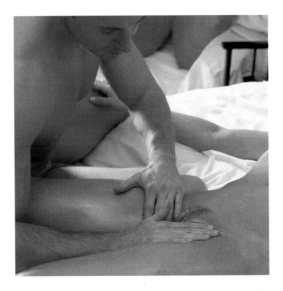

Talking lube

If you are a woman with a new partner, discuss the joys of almond oil before you get to the bedroom, so there's not an awkward pause while you make explanations that could ruin the mood. Talk about it on an occasion when you feel close but are not yet ready to embark on the sexual side of your relationship, explaining that erotic massage with plenty of oil is one of your favourite things. Then when it comes to the time for it, there'll be no embarrassment.

If you're already in an established relationship there should be no shyness about discussing lubrication, but you may need to reassure your partner that dryness is quite normal and you haven't gone off him.

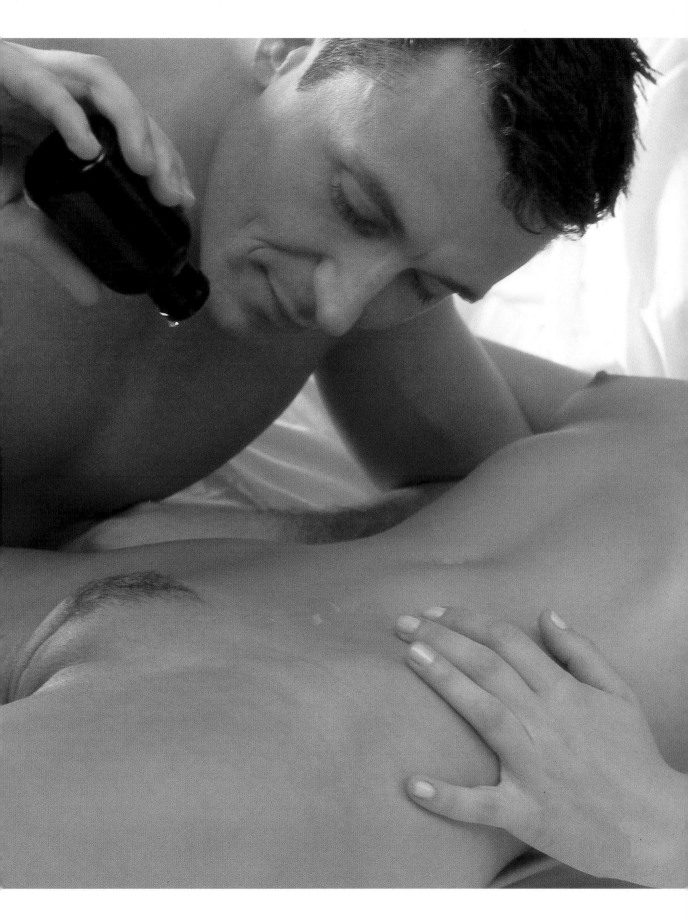

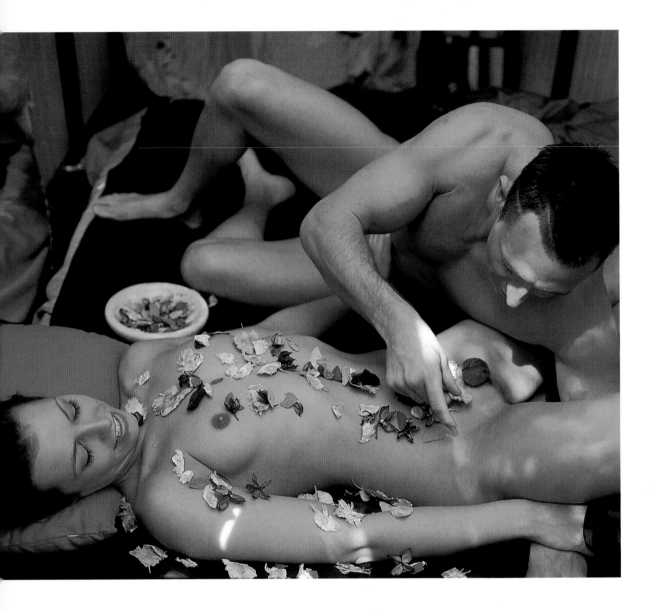

Fragrance

Did you know that the smell of cinnamon buns increases the flow of blood to the penis? An American neurologist discovered this in laboratory experiments. He also found that wafts of lavender, pumpkin pie, liquorice and doughnuts can induce stronger erections. Probably all these warm, sweet, homely smells remind American men of their childhood and make them feel happy and secure. The aromas of fresh flowers, baking bread or cakes, ripe peaches and apricots, furniture polish and clean sheets can all enliven the sense of smell, which is powerfully connected to memory and emotion, and provide a relaxing background to lovemaking.

The scent of love

The natural perfume of a clean woman is called her *cassolette* – French for perfume box. Inhale it from her hair, skin, armpits, genitals and the clothes she has been wearing. The natural smell of both sexes forms a strong part in sexual attraction – marriage counsellors know that an aversion to a partner's smell is one thing no amount of therapy can overturn.

Use your lover's smell to excite you – bury your head in an old T-shirt before you meet. Or use it to calm and comfort you after a row. The smell will remind you of why you are together.

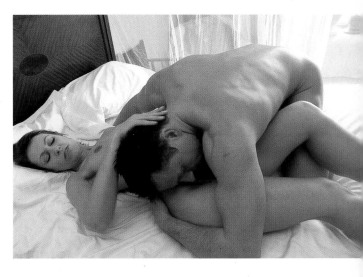

Rose petals

Buy her roses, or pick them from the garden. Then drop the petals one by one on her naked body. Sniff their fragrance – lick round them lovingly and press them into her skin with your tongue. Finally, make love with the petals crushed between you.

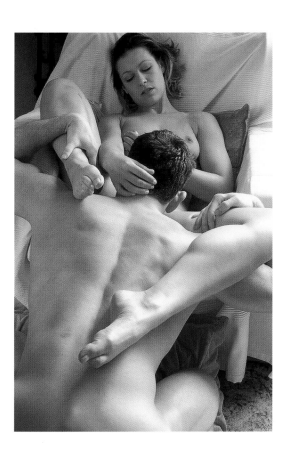

Aromatherapy oils for erotic massage

Francincense A spicy woody aroma known for its aphrodisiac properties. It relaxes, rejuvenates and enlivens the emotions.

Geranium A floral scent that has a relieving effect on anxiety.

Jasmine Rich, exotic and sensual, this lifts the mood and is highly regarded for its aphrodisiac effect.

Juniper A woody scent that is good for stimulating and relaxing. Relieves stress and fatigue.

Patchouli A seductive Oriental aroma and the base of many heavy perfumes. Redolent of the harem.

Ylang ylang An exotic, Far-Eastern scent that is used as a love potion. Very effective both as a stimulant and a sedative.

Body piercing

Rings and jewels can be worn on any part of the body that can be pierced – not only the ears, nose and eyebrows, but also through the tongue, nipples, navel, penis, scrotum and labia. Erotic piercing has been popular in many cultures for centuries. Queen Victoria's consort Prince Albert is attributed with the invention of the penis ring named after him, though he is said to have tied a cord through it to his leg to stop involuntary nocturnal erections. Some couples today wear gold rings in their genitals – through the labia and scrotum – instead of wearing wedding rings on their fingers.

Caution

Piercing can be dangerous. Not only is it painful at the time, the pain may last months while the wound heals and infection can easily set in. Many people are allergic to the metals used in piercing needles or in jewellery. Some piercings may result in permanent nerve damage.

Always choose a licensed practitioner, preferably one who has been personally recommended to you. Wash the wound daily with a recommended antiseptic, rotating the ring or bar to keep the hole open, until it has healed.

Erotic rings

Rings in the labia don't increase erotic sensation – they are worn simply for their looks. Sometimes rings on either side of the vulva are used to pull back the labia for sex.

According to Arab tradition, rings in the scrotum prevent the testicles from ever rising back into the body.

In the South Pacific, a ring called a *guiche* is placed at the point where the scrotum joins the perineum, in front of the anus. If correctly placed, it is said to intensify and prolong orgasms when gently pulled.

The Southeast Asian *ampallang* is a rod that pierces horizontally through the glans of the penis above the urethra. It is said to increase firmness during erection. Sometimes the rod has a ring around it that encircles the glans. Bead-like protuberances on the ring are designed to stimulate the vulva and clitoris during sex.

Nipple rings were worn by Roman centurions, who used them as fixings for their cloaks. Victorian women also wore them to simulate their nipples under their clothes.

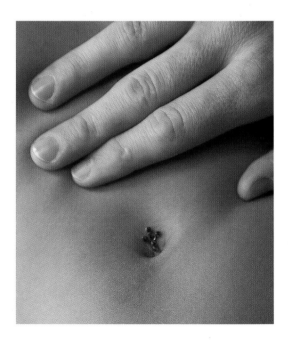

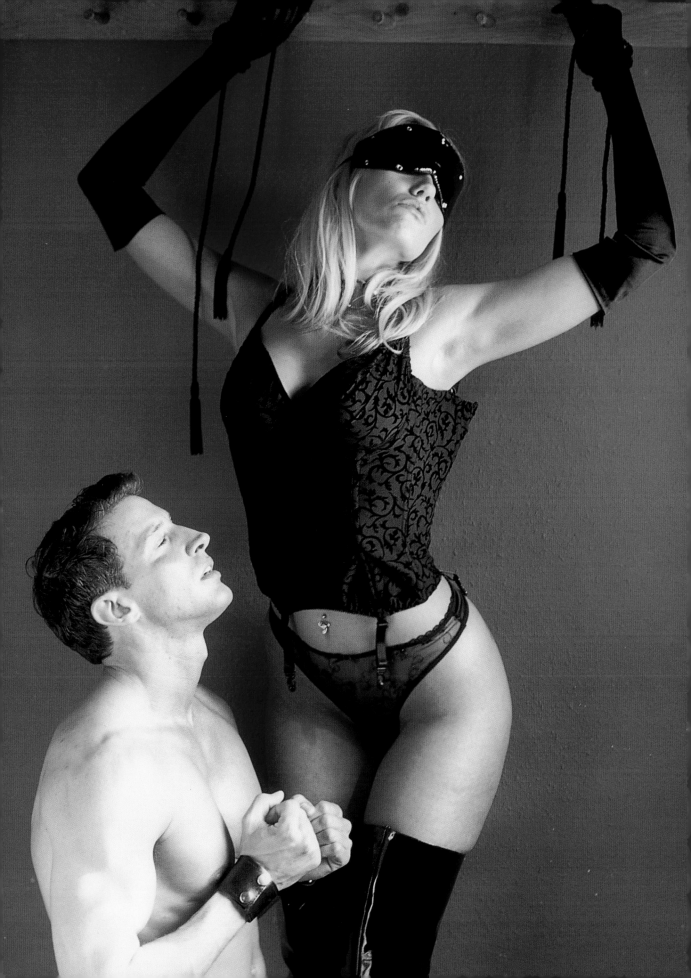

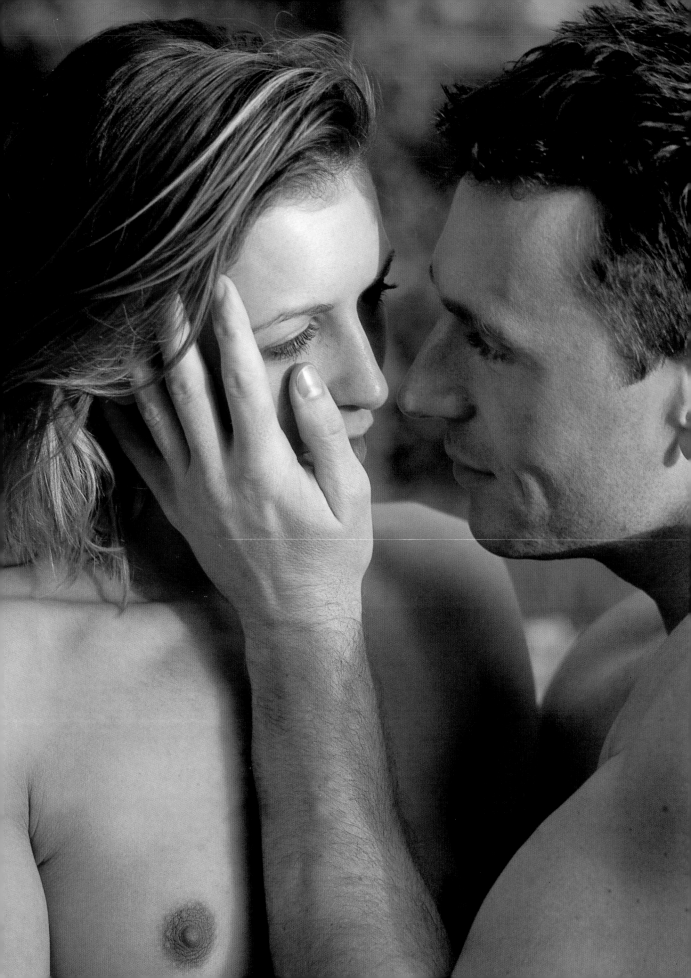

Aphrodisiacs

The body's most important sex organ is the brain – and when it comes to aphrodisiacs you can be sure it's almost always in the mind. Canadian researchers recently tested the drug yohimbine, extracted from the yohimbe plant, which is used by the Bantu people of Africa as a male aphrodisiac. They found that 42 per cent of a group of men with erection difficulties responded well to the treatment – but so did 28 per cent of the control group, who were all given sugar pill placebos!

Sex and drugs?

Everyone knows that alcohol loosens the tongue and the inhibitions – but though it enlivens at first, it's basically a depressant. A little too much and you'll be drowsy – more than that and the urge and ability will leave altogether. Go for quality not quantity – share one good bottle of wine with an excellent meal and intimate conversation to put you in the mood for love.

One survey conducted in Italy found that while men reported increased sexual satisfaction with Viagra, their partners were not impressed. If you try Viagra don't forget to make your partner feel that you want her – not just your own satisfaction.

Recreational drugs, like alcohol, induce a chemical high followed by an emotional low, though dreamy cannabis encourages sleep, not sex. Ask yourselves whether it's sex you want, or each other. It can be a lonely and alienating experience if you get the feeling your partner's deriving their pleasure from taking a drug instead of from being with you.

And still on the subject of drugs – did you know that smoking can seriously damage your sex life? It's not just the wheezing and bad breath – nicotine reduces the production of nitric oxide, the body's main chemical messenger that triggers the pumping of blood to the penis. Another good reason for giving up the weed.

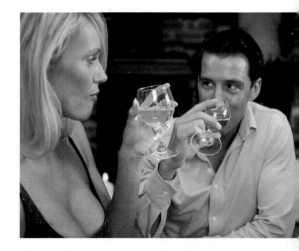

The power of thought

Whether it's oysters, caviar or wild yams, if you like it, believe in it and are in the right mood for it to work, then work it surely will. Give thanks for the positive power of thought. Something that often does the trick is dark chocolate. It stimulates the brain to produce phenylethylamine, a chemical that is triggered when we fall in love. So putting a chocolate on your lover's pillow will send a sexy message... Try sharing a chocolate kiss. You can even buy chocolate-flavoured body paint, so why wait until you get to heaven...

The no-hands massage

Move on to a no-hands massage after a full erotic massage (see pages 10-29), or incorporate some of these techniques into any steamy sex session. Perhaps the ultimate arousing experience is a massage using only the tongue. Oil your partner's body first so your tongue doesn't dry out – use plenty of oil on hairy skin – and lubricate as you go with generous amounts of saliva. Many people find sucking and slurping noises turn them on, so don't hold back!

Where to start

The chest, belly, upper thighs, back and buttocks are the main areas to focus on, and some people also adore having their toes and fingers noisily sucked one by one.

On the back, lick in a firm rippling motion all down the spine, then work lavishly on the buttocks, pushing them up and apart to create tension on the genitals and tugging at the flesh with your lips to suck and lick. Finish by nuzzling the inner thighs and tickling them lightly with your tongue. On the torso, start by probing the navel with your tongue, then circle round and round the belly with lapping strokes in a clockwise direction. Draw a firm wavy line with your tongue right up the centre of the chest, then follow the lines of the ribs in a zigzag in and out to the sides. Circle the breasts and finish by flicking and sucking the nipples.

More hot massage ideas

Massage with the vulva Straddle your partner and massage his torso with your vulva – apply plenty of oil first and this will be a delicious experience for both of you.

Hair massage You can do this even if you have fairly short hair – but don't oil your partner's body first. Lean over his or her torso and brush it up and down and round and round with your trailing (or short and bushy) locks. This is a lovely soothing experience especially with eyes closed.

Nipple massage Lean over your partner and massage him with your nipples, in broad strokes up and down his body, or gyrating and drawing tantalizing circles on his skin. Massage his penis between your breasts – without touching it with your hands.

Foot massage Sit above your partner with legs dangling, and trace patterns on his well oiled body with your big toes. In China women learned how to pleasure their partners by gripping the penis between the soles of their feet...

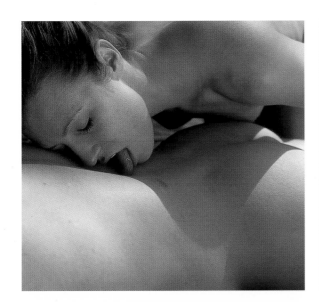
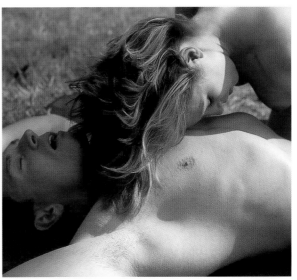
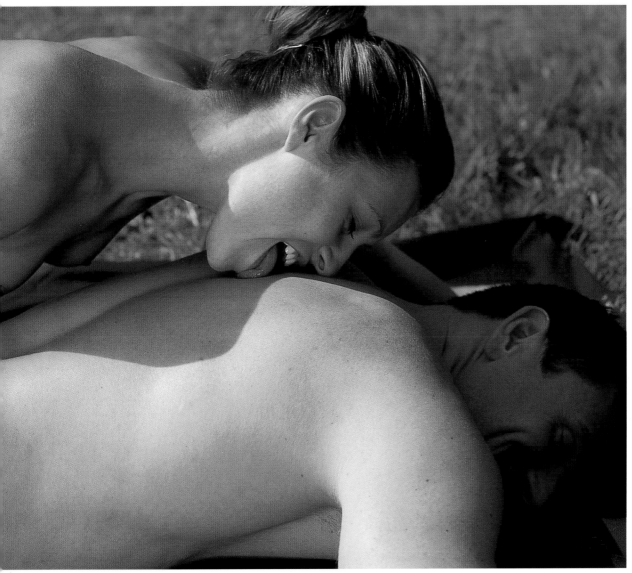

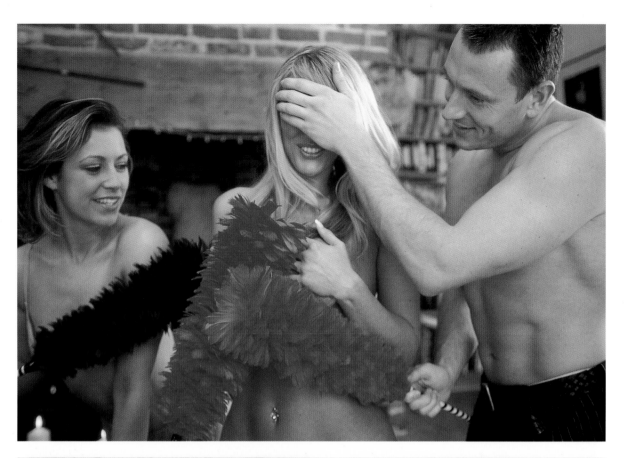

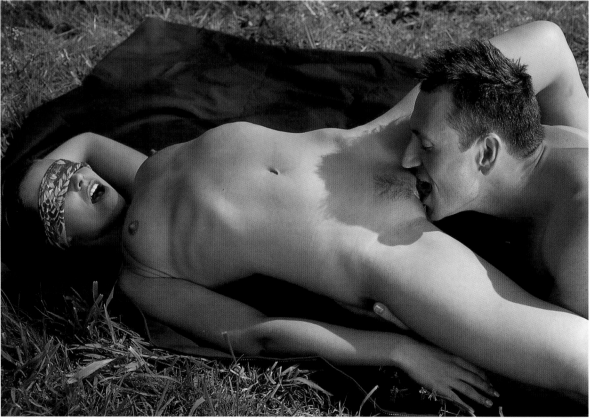

Blindfold sensations

Blindfold your lover to make his sense of touch more acute, then experiment with different sensations – texture, temperature, pressure – on various parts of his body. Keep it slow and full of surprises. Discover which parts of the body are most sensitive to each mystery stimulant – get him to describe what he's feeling and guess what's happening to him...

Stimulating sensations

Cool treat Ice cream and fruit sorbets are edible coolants that you can use imaginatively and deliciously on your partner's body.

Ice Try cooling your partner down with ice during a sexual massage. The forehead is an obvious place to start, but you can also doodle patterns around the nipples with an ice cube, then circle it tantalizingly around the belly, over the inner thighs and across the genitals. (Never use dry ice, as it will stick to and burn the skin.)

More ice Try giving your partner oral sex with crushed ice in your mouth. During fellatio this technique is sometimes used to delay orgasm.

Hot air Heat up your mouth with a warm drink before you go down on your partner.

Hot compress Fit an inflatable bath pillow filled with hot water under his neck and place miniature hot water bottles at strategic points on his body. Or use little 'beanbags' of wheat heated up in the microwave. Now doodle round the beanbags with a feather, an ice cube or warm spoons dipped in oil.

Fur Let the animal inside him loose by stroking his skin with fur, real or fake – it feels especially lovely on the chest and belly.

Rhythm Use the tasselled drumsticks from a snare drum to whip up a rhythm on his back or buttocks, or try an egg whisk made of pliant twigs, or even the tassels sold as curtain tie-backs.

Feathers Try stroking your lover's skin with a feather or a boa made of swansdown.

Marbles Massage his stomach and chest with a handful of marbles, rolling them in small clockwise circles.

Rice Shower him with rice, or pour it in a stream all down his spine. Drift confetti on to his cheeks, neck and genitals.

Sweet sensation Dribble warm honey on to his erect penis and suck it off.

Gel Use a lovely squidgy gel – sold as a moisturizing face mask – for rubbing into nipples and genitals. Slather it on really thickly, paying thorough attention to inner thighs and perineum before you move on to scrotum and penis.

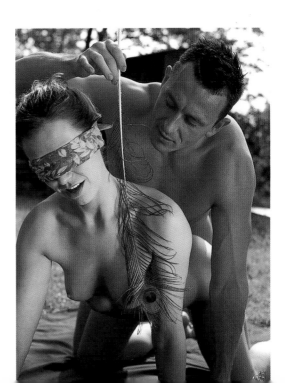

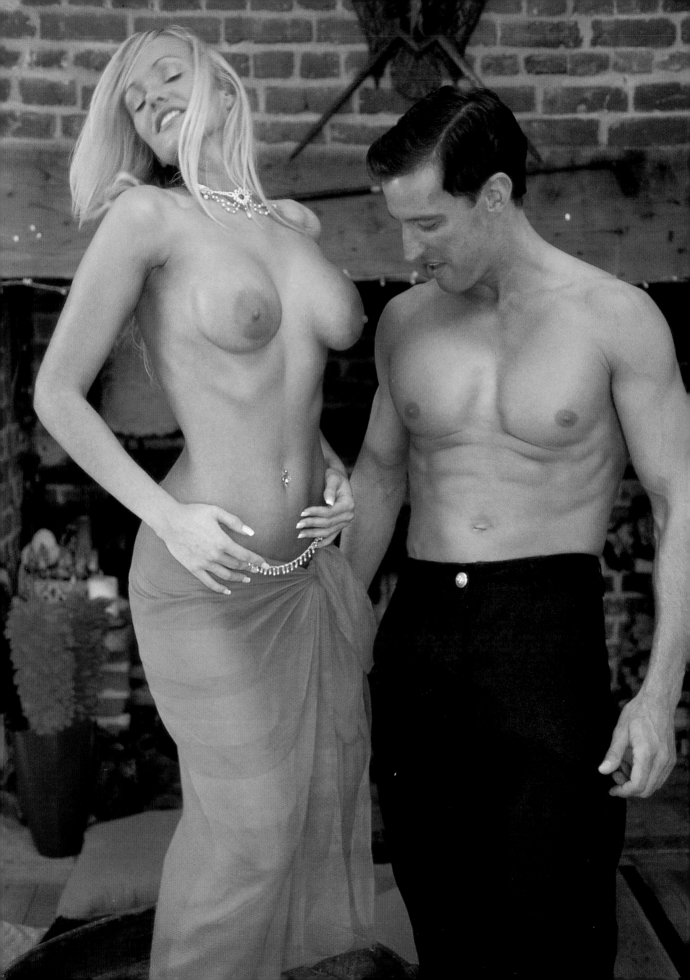

Belly dancing

In the East, the gently rounded belly of a woman is one of her most sensual attributes, appreciated to the full in the skilful and sensuous art of belly dancing. The smoothly undulating hips suggest the burning passions of the harem, and in addition to its sexual fascination, belly dancing is good for you.

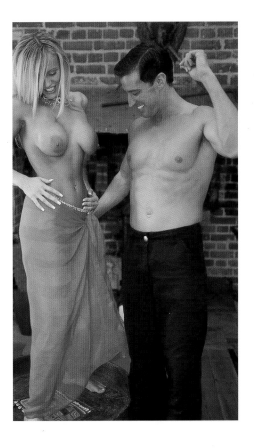

The belly roll

One of the key movements of belly dancing, this relaxes and sensitizes the whole body. It imitates the contractions of labour and gives sexual confidence. Place both thumbs on your navel with your palms flat on your lower belly. Push the lower belly out, then pull it in and up as far as you can, pulling in your diaphragm too. Now push your diaphragm out and let your belly roll down and out. Begin slowly, then repeat the sequence, speeding up to a steady rhythm.

A variation, the belly flutter, concentrates on the diaphragm. For this movement, either hold your breath, or keep your mouth open and pant. Contract the diaphragm and then push it out. Repeat slowly at first, then build up speed until your belly is vibrating fast.

The hip roll

Stand relaxed and upright, with your arms out to the sides, palms facing up. Push the right hip out to the right side. Push the pelvis forward as far as you can and roll your hips over to the left. Push the pelvis back to the rear, sticking your bottom out. Straighten your knees, then roll the hips to the right. Carry on rolling the hips in a large smooth circle, as if you were swinging a hula hoop around your waist.

The benefits

An awareness of the belly as the centre of the self gives confidence and solidity, it improves the posture, eases stress and lifts depression, as well as exercising and toning many of the muscles used in sex. Above all, it gives you a sense of vitality and a belief in your own erotic power. Try the exercises here, then make up your own variations. Add some silk scarves and jewels, dramatize your eyes with kohl and prepare to amaze your lover.

Heavy petting

Get imaginative and invent new ways of having sex without intercourse to rediscover the steamy days of your youth. Heavy petting stops short of genital-to-genital contact (originally as a contraceptive measure or to keep her virginity intact) – but anything else goes, creating an almost unbearably heady mix of frustration and excitement.

Sex without intercourse

If you don't like menstrual blood, but she feels particularly raunchy when she has a period, this could be one solution. It's also great to try if your sex life has grown tired or predictable and has become just a one-track route to orgasm. There's certainly no pressure to perform if intercourse is off the menu.

Keep your clothes on

Start fully clothed, then loosen or remove clothing as required, but agree in advance that she will keep her panties on and there won't be any penetration. Move through a variety of sex positions (this is a good way to practice new moves for the real thing on another occasion). The friction of his penis against her vulva might well give her an orgasm, but don't carry on so long that it makes him sore.

Between the breasts

Many men fantasize about coming between a woman's breasts. Best done with him sitting in a chair with legs splayed, and his lover kneeling in front of him. She begins by caressing his penis with her breasts and tickling the glans with her nipples, then squeezes him between her breasts and works up and down, holding the base of the penis with one hand and pressing her breasts together with the other. Add oil and work with passion. A smaller woman can try masturbating him against her breasts while caressing them with her other hand.

Between the thighs

The woman clenches her partner's penis between her thighs at the very top – in either the missionary position or with her lying on her back or crouching on all-fours. If he ejaculates, it's very easy for sperm to get transferred to the vagina, so note this is not a good position for contraception.

Mutual masturbation

This is a delicious way of satisfying each other, whether it's during heavy petting or part of a full lovemaking session.

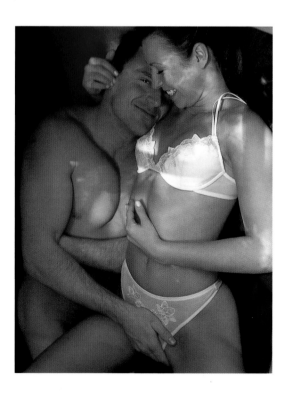

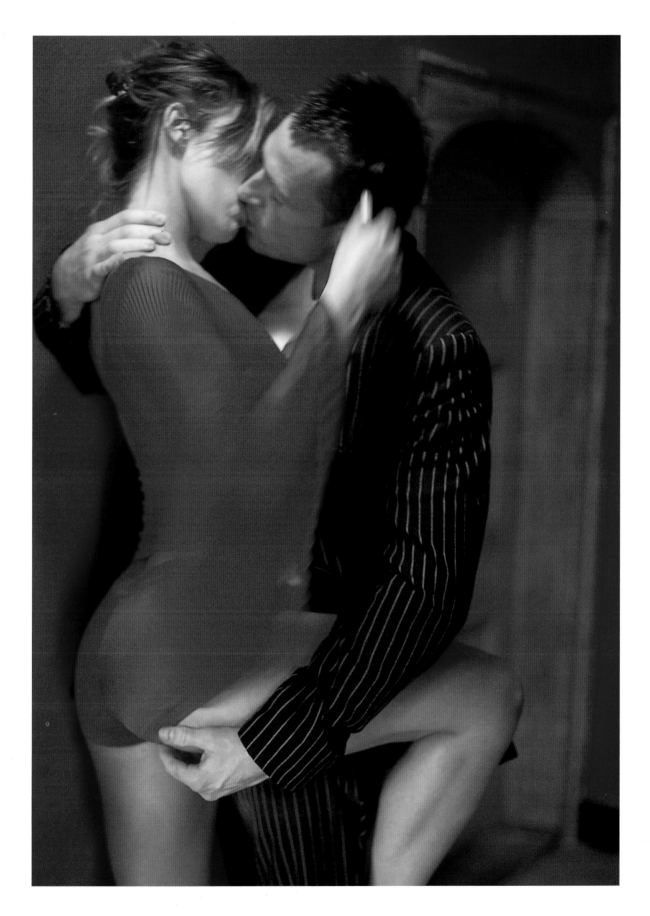

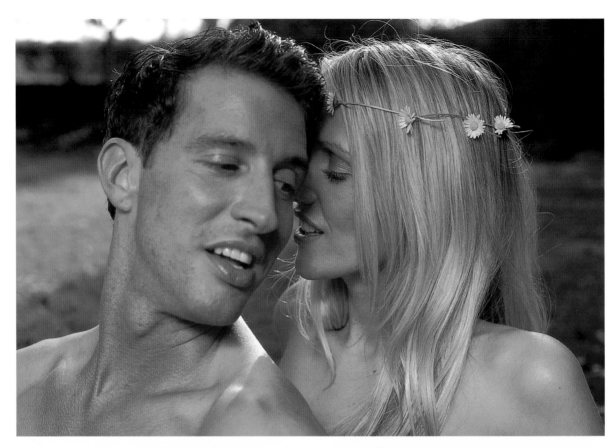

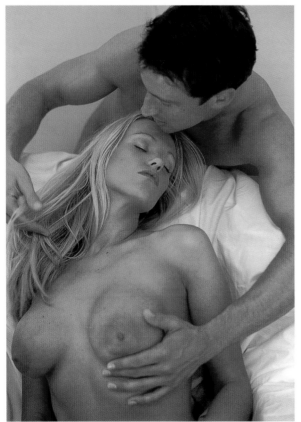

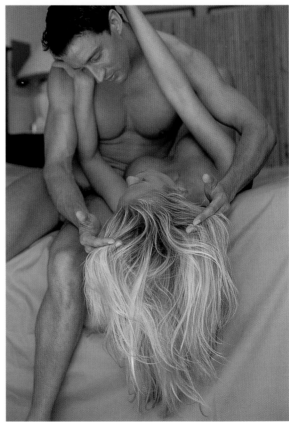

Hair

The hair has always held sexual magic. Lovers once exchanged locks of hair and in some cultures the bride and groom are shampooed in the same basin at their wedding, then their hair is twisted together in one strand to unite the pair for life. In ancient India a courtesan would seduce a new patron with an erotic hair dance, rubbing her hair with perfumed oils, then swinging it loose with passionate movements of her head. Hair symbolised sexual energy for men too, and cutting it meant castration. (Think of Samson.) To this day many Muslim men keep their hair long and wrapped in a turban to preserve its vital essences.

Follow the *Kama Sutra*

Students of the *Kama Sutra* learned the arts of beautifying the hair by colouring it with henna and dressing it in braids, chaplets and topknots of flowers. While the hair on the head was celebrated, men shaved their beards and both sexes removed all body hair.

Ideas from an ancient Indian love text

1. One of the best ways of kindling hot desire in a woman is at the time of rising, softly to hold and handle her hair...

2. The man encloses her hair between his two palms behind her head, at the same time kissing her lower lip...

3. 'the dragon's turn' is when the man, excited by the approaching prospect of sexual congress, amorously seizes the hind knot of the woman's hair, at the same time closely embracing her. This is done in a standing position and is one of the most exciting acts of love play...

4. 'Holding the crest-hair of love' is when, during the act of copulation, the man holds with both hands his partner's hair above her ears, whist she does the same to him, and both exchange frequent kisses on the mouth...

Try this

Dress your hair for love. Make a simple daisy chain or a garland of ivy leaves or vine leaves.

Sex without pubic hair feels closer still – more naked, more vulnerable. So make a ritual of shaping your pubic hair or removing it entirely. This is something you can do together. If shaving irritates, use a depilatory cream.

Sexual activity makes a man's beard grow. It can feel like sandpaper on your lover's tender skin, so freshly, smoothly shaved is best for sex.

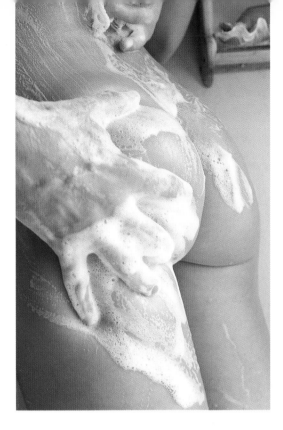

Showers

From schooldays on, sex and showers are strongly connected in the mind. The seductive discipline of showering after sport starts around puberty, when boys and girls are curious to observe each others' naked bodies and compare sexual development as they rush shyly into the showers and are forced to soap themselves in full view.

Steam and soap

In adult life, showers provide a natural environment for sex. Check out the erotic descriptions of gay sex in Alan Hollinghurst's *The Swimming Pool Library*, where the showers at the pool are always full of lithe hunks soaping their throbbing erections. The shower is a favourite place for a man to go all the way with masturbation, relieving all the tensions of the day.

Things to do in the shower

Watch him At the climax of a blue movie the male star withdraws so he can be watched as he ejaculates on to his partner's belly, breasts or face. Sit mesmerized in a chair while your partner puts on a fine show for you in the shower.

Water massage With the temperature just right and the shower full on, use the hose to give your partner a water massage. A bath hose is best for massaging her genitals – and some women love it so much that they come as the water gently needles their vulva and clitoris.

Lathering up Use plenty of soap or shower gel to make each other hot and slippery. Concentrate on getting the genitals into a real lather, then when neither can wait any longer, he picks her up and she grips round his waist with her legs as he enters her. She can support her back against the wall of the shower as he holds her buttocks. Let the hot water rain down on you as you make love.

Golden showers The shower is the place to play a favourite game of childhood with an erotic twist – golden showers. Go wild and do it all over each other. Try turning the shower off when you start to flow, so you can feel the warmth of each other's urine. He can put his hand between her legs and she can play with his penis, pointing it at her belly and breasts.

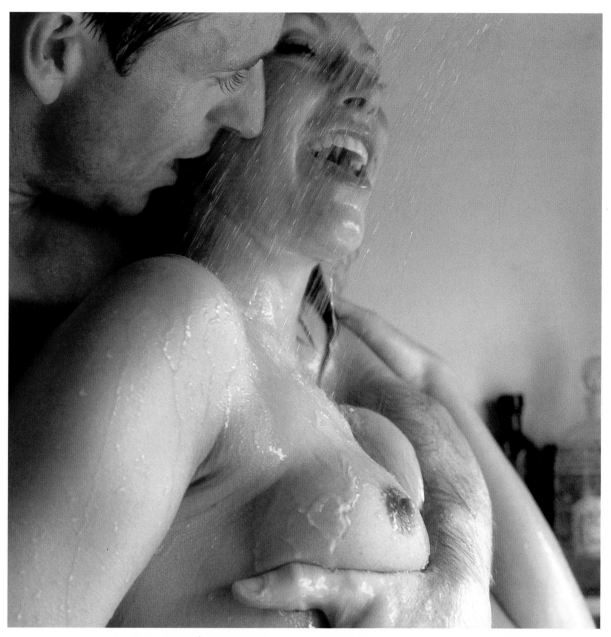

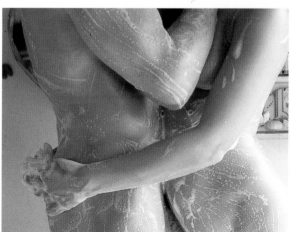

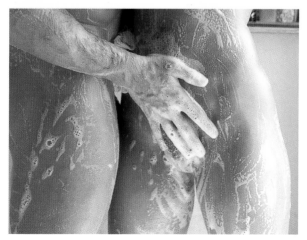

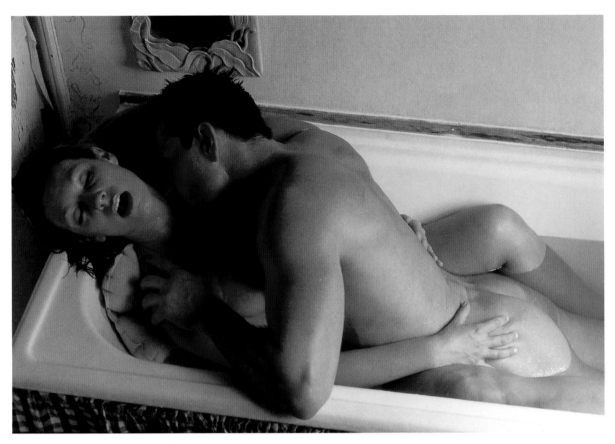

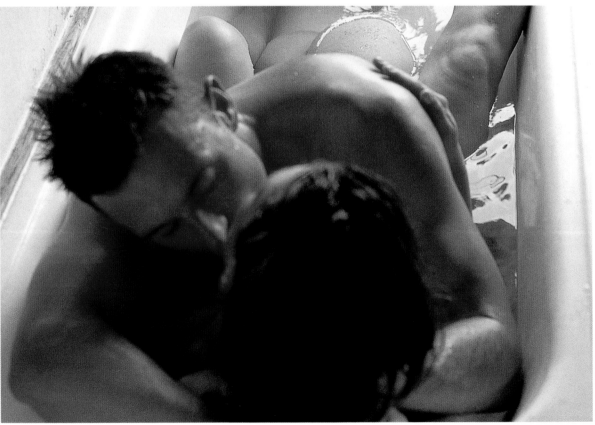

Water babies

Ever made love standing up to your chests in the sea? This is a good way to relieve the frustration caused by rubbing suntan lotion into your partner's sizzling hot, near-naked body on the beach. To watching sunbathers you just look like a couple kissing with your arms around each other, but under the water her legs are round his waist and something more exciting's going on...

Making waves

There's nothing quite like making love in a rowing boat under a curtain of dreamily trailing willows. All your movements are emphasised by the rocking of the boat, giving a delicious sensation of freedom. Things to remember: take a picnic. Find a secluded spot and moor the boat securely (very important!). Take plenty of cushions and a rug, in case of chilly breezes or stray passers-by. A perfect occasion to wear a full skirt with nothing underneath it.

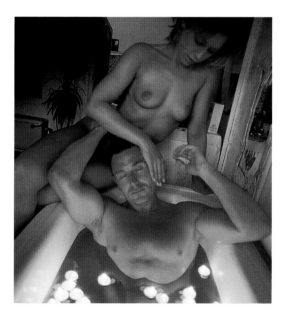

Bath time tips

Make bath time something special. In the evening, add candles, music, luxurious oils or rose petals sprinkled on the water. Or suggest a bath in the middle of the day as a surprise to completely lift your mood. Add masses of foam.

1. Water, paradoxically, is drying. Apply plenty of lube before you immerse yourselves.

2. Combine bath time with a steamy mutual pubic hairdressing session.

3. Give your partner an underwater massage with creamy soap. Pay special attention to areas of tension around the neck and shoulders, so he or she is completely relaxed before you start to soap the genitals. Be extremely thorough here, diligently exploring every millimetre of the pelvic area with tantalisingly slippery, gently probing fingers.

4. Be inventive with sex positions to overcome the limitations of the tub. It's good for mutual masturbation. Then try woman sitting on top as man reclines. Then she can lie back too – rock gently into each other – try not to cause a flood. Or she can sit on his lap, facing the taps.

5. Don't forget to keep warm – top up frequently with hot water.

6. Afterwards, go straight to bed, still wet but wrapped tightly in huge towels. It's a really relaxing way to fall asleep together.

Do it al fresco

There's something truly erotic about sex in the open air – nowhere else will you feel so naked, so spontaneous, or so natural. There is nothing quite like the caress of sunshine and warm breezes as bare skin meets bare skin, or the sighing of the wind in the leaves, and the reflections of clouds in your lover's eyes. The changing natural light on the textures of skin and hair, the rich scent of earth and crushed grass, and the feeling of space all around heighten the senses and add to the sensation of wonder. Sex outside powerfully connects with the rhythms of nature, and brings an exquisite vulnerability. The possibility of discovery by others is part of the thrill.

What to take

Take a blanket or, even better, a double sleeping bag – having your pelvis scraped against twigs and stones can make passion wear thin!

Note that haystacks are soft and smell wonderful, but stacks of straw bales are prickly.

For a longer session, take a tent (a two-person tent that erects itself) – then you can fall asleep afterwards, even in the rain.

No tent? Take gauzy curtains or filmy muslin to hang in the trees and make a temple of love.

If it's hot, go armed with water sprays to cool each other down, or water pistols, or water bombs.

Don't forget the mosquito repellent.

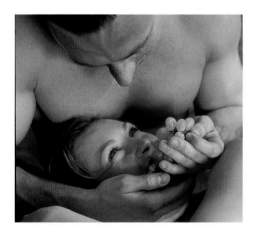

And where?

Find a clearing in a wood.

Find a tree with a low branch that the woman can bend over, and make love standing.

The beach – go skinny dipping first; later have a barbecue under the stars.

The back garden by moonlight. Will the neighbours see? Do you care?

Lovers' picnic

Take a picnic you can eat with your fingers, and include delicious aphrodisiac foods that you can feed each other. Try the following:

- Asparagus spears rolled in prosciutto
- Prawns with chilli dip
- Fresh fruit: figs, grapes, strawberries, slices of melon to bite into and let the juices run
- A bottle of chilled white wine or champagne
- Dark chocolate

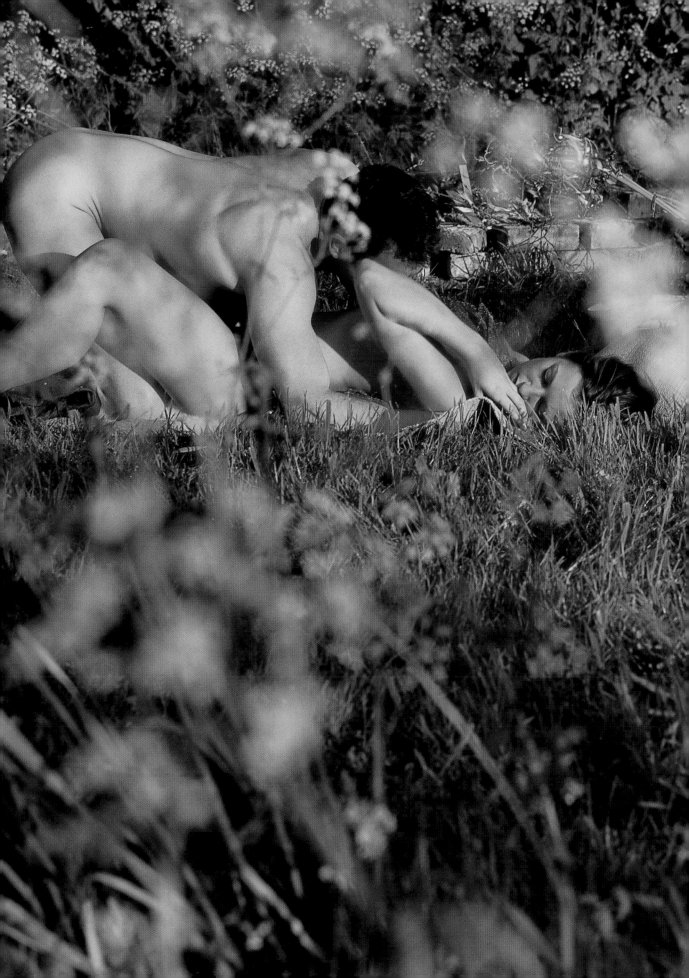

Cupboard love

Sometimes when you're overtaken by lust among a crowd of people, the only place you'll find any privacy is the broom closet – or the bathroom. If you're at a party choose your moment to slip into the bathroom together. In a public place it's a little trickier, but that's all part of the fun. Angles of deep penetration are good for fast furious sex when anticipation is high and there's no scope for foreplay.

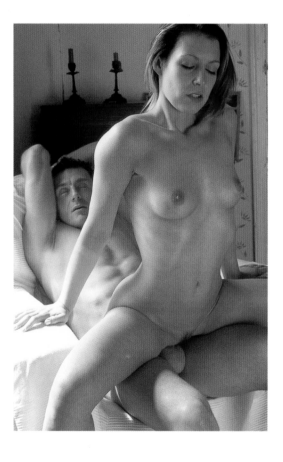

Six positions for fast sex in a cramped space

1. The man sits on whatever is available. The woman straddles his lap, facing him. She controls the pace as she moves vigorously up and down on him, supporting herself with her feet on the floor and her arms round his neck.

2. The man sits. The woman faces away from him as she lowers herself on to him. This is a position of deep penetration. The man can help her move by holding her firmly at the waist as she bounces up and down.

3. The woman leans over a wash basin. He enters her standing from behind. A good position for female orgasm as the penis stimulates the front wall of the vagina.

4. The woman sits on the edge of the stairs. The man kneels in front of her. She opens her legs and wraps them round him as he enters her. He pulls her towards him, she leans back and he supports her with his arms round her back.

5. The man stands. His partner stands on the loo facing him. He supports her by joining his hands round her back and she clasps him round the neck. She lowers herself on to him, wrapping her legs around his back.

6. Another standing position. This time the man holds the woman's buttocks to support her weight and she leans back against the wall as he thrusts into her. In a small cubicle she can rest her feet on the opposite wall.

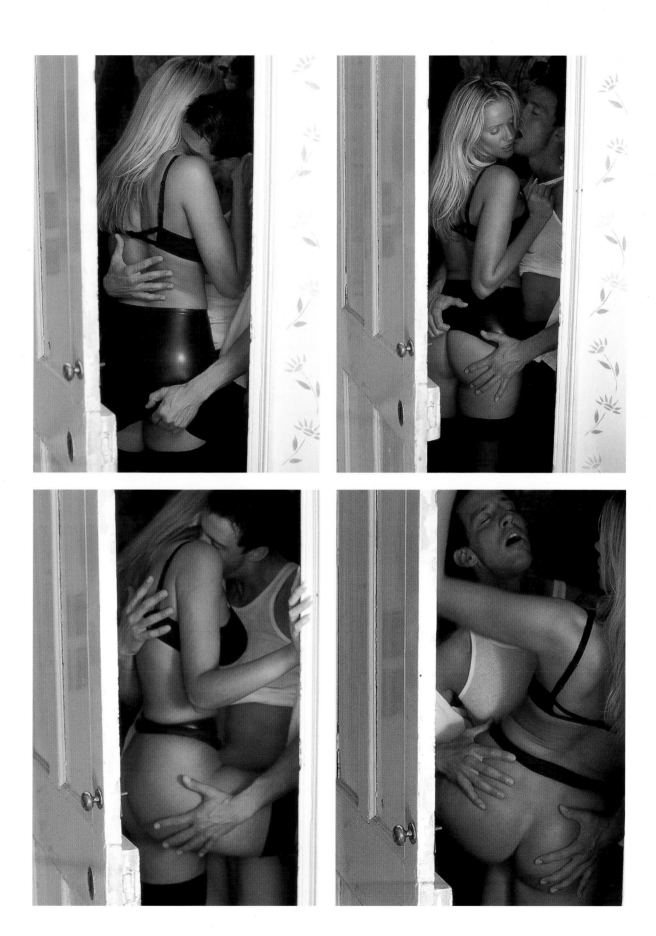

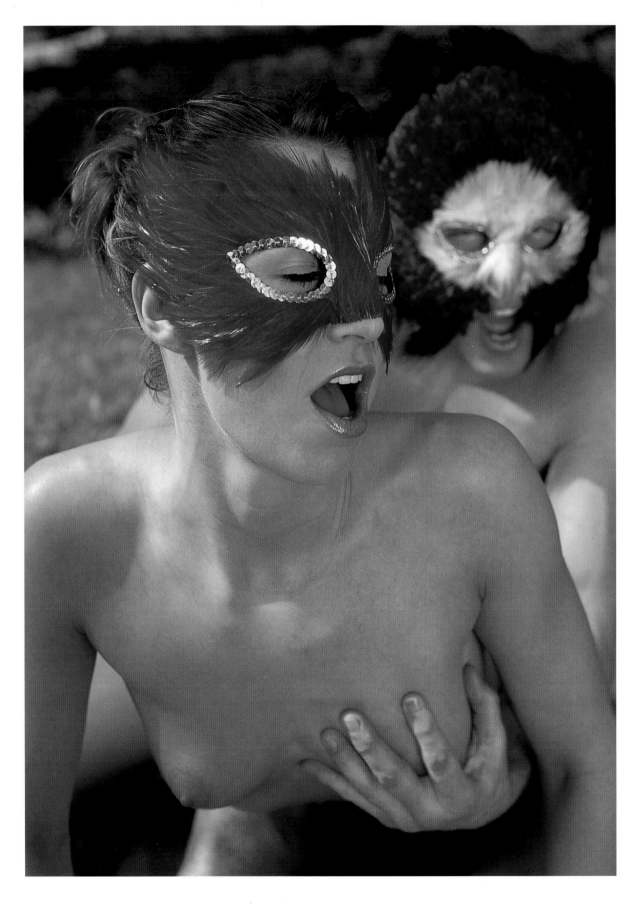

Fantasy

Most of us start to learn about sex through childhood games, but in adulthood it's easy to let the pressure to do it right make us forget that sex is all about playing together. So what sexy games do you play in your daydreams? Lots of people have fantasies about their current partners that involve a surprising shift, such as sex in an unusual location or costume. It may feel daft to talk to her about it, but imagine how exciting it would be if after years of dreaming of your partner answering the door to you naked, she actually did it!

Playing games

Fantasies are worth sharing – or swapping for one of hers – and acting them out could make your sex life take off like a rocket. But be careful about revealing fantasies that involve a third person – your partner may not be so keen to hear that you fancy your neighbour. Of course, it's understood that having a fantasy about someone doesn't mean you're looking for an opportunity to get into bed with them in real life, but if you want to make your partner happy, steer clear of anything that might rebound on you in the future. Try these games for starters...

Stranger Arrange to meet your partner in a bar. When you get there you barely recognize her as she has transformed her appearance and is wearing completely different clothes and make-up. She pretends that she does not know you. Your job is to chat her up and take her home – she plays hard to get...

Casting couch Arrange to meet your partner at a hotel. One of you is the movie mogul and the other is the up-and-coming star looking for a part. Over dinner the plot of the film is discussed and the actor is grilled. The mogul then invites him or her into the bedroom for an in-depth consultation...

Fancy dress Go where the imagination takes you – anything from royal regalia to grass skirts. The drama and erotic mystery of a masked ball has always offered the opportunity for the sexual alter ego to run amok – hold a fancy dress party and see what happens...

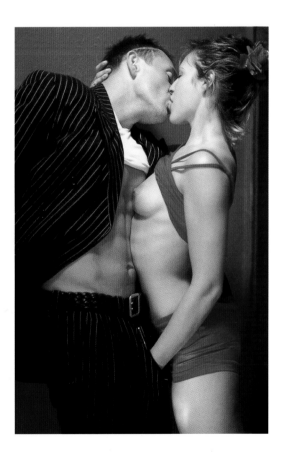

Doctors and nurses In a new twist on a childhood game, try playing at sexologists. The sexologist is there to study the patient's sexual response – so anything goes...

Customs officer and smuggler Involves a uniform, a body search, smuggled goods and bribery with sexual favours...

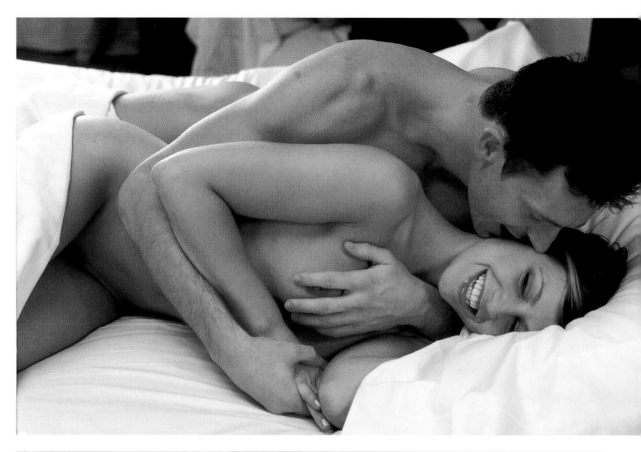

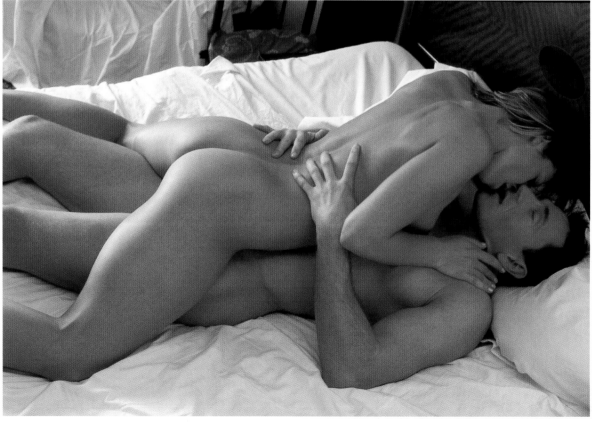

Sex talk

The sounds of sex have their own excitement – the sighs and moans, the grunts and groans of satisfaction – it's a terrific turn-on to know that what you're doing is blowing your partner's mind. And lots of people enjoy the music their bodies make together – the sounds of licking, sucking and lapping, and even vaginal farts. But sex talk is what drives some people really wild. Both men and women love to hear their partners heat up and let rip verbally – some relish everything from whispered endearments and encouragements to a crude running commentary and shouted obscenities.

Why is filthy language a turn-on?

Simply, because it's forbidden – so the more unusual it is for your partner to use four-letter words and language that makes the air go blue, the more exciting it's likely to be. To express what usually takes place only inside your head is to break down yet another inhibition and release more pent-up libido you didn't know you had.

The sad thing about obscenities in many languages is that we use forbidden sex words to express anger and as insults. In less-repressed cultures, sex words are used for sex. So a Swede might shout something about yellow snow and a Native American might call someone a failed horse-breaker, but neither would use 'fuck' except in pleasure. Try using words as they were originally intended and feel their erotic power.

Caution: don't introduce sex talk the first time you get into bed with someone – some prefer silence and some find it offensive and threatening.

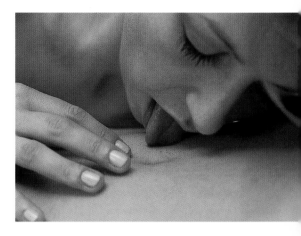

Say it to me

During long slow thrusting a man can whisper his secret lusts and desires for her into his partner's ear. He can tell her what he's planning to do to her next, then do it.

Tell your partner what feels wonderful and how wonderful it feels while he's actually doing it, and it will rouse his passion even more. It's a fantastic ego-boost that can spur your lover on to more imaginative and longer-lasting sex.

Tell your partner your fantasies during mutual masturbation – especially erotic daydreams that feature him or her having sex with someone else. This is a very good way to work yourselves up into a very steamy lather.

Telephone sex. When you and your lover are apart and long for sex, let the telephone bring you together. Detailed descriptions of what you are both doing and feeling are the next best things to being there.

Je t'aime. Lots of people like to be talked to in bed in a foreign language – whether they understand it or not.

Reading in bed

Bedtime stories have been around ever since Scheherazade escaped the death sentence by relating one thousand and one erotic tales to her Arabian king. Reading stories in bed to your lover recreates the intimate warmth and security of the childhood bedtime story, and you can add the endings that won't send you to sleep!

Tell and kiss

Try this. Each of you keeps a private collection of erotic books and stories on your own bedside table. On story night, take it in turns to read them aloud, then see where the imagination takes you. Or shut the book at a crucial point in the story and ask your partner to relate what happens next. Another time, try creating a sexy narrative of your own. Take it in turns – each of you adds a word that brings the story nearer to its orgasmic climax, and both of you try to keep it going as long as possible. You may make some interesting discoveries about each other's secret desires without even trying...

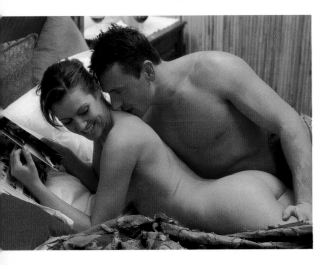

What happens next?

1. Eunuchs disguised as females keep their desires secret and lead the life of shampooers. Under the pretence of shampooing, a eunuch embraces and draws towards himself the thighs of the man he is shampooing, touching the joints of his thighs. Then, if he finds the lingam of the man erect....

2. My lips fired and emboldened him, and now, glancing my eyes toward that part of his dress which covered the essential object of enjoyment, I plainly discovered the swell and commotion there, and as I was now too far advanced to stop....

3. Pear Blossom poured wine for Lady Ping and her guest and left the pair to their guilty pleasures. Believing themselves alone, how quickly the lovers undressed one another with urgent fingers. But what is this? Pear Blossom the sly one has made a hole in the paper of the wall so she can spy upon the lovers at their games....

4. The sea and the sun had rendered her blonder than ever and her mouth was the same pink as the pink of her open sex. So that Sir Stephen could see every bit of her, O took care to flex Jacqueline's knees and to keep her legs wide apart. The shutters were drawn and the room was almost dark. For almost an hour Jacqueline moaned under O's caresses, and finally....

5. Whilst our lips clung together, his hand slowly, imperceptibly, unbuttoned my trousers, and stealthily slipped within, turning every obstacle in its way instinctively aside, then it lay hold of my hard, stiff, and aching phallus, which was glowing like a burning coal....

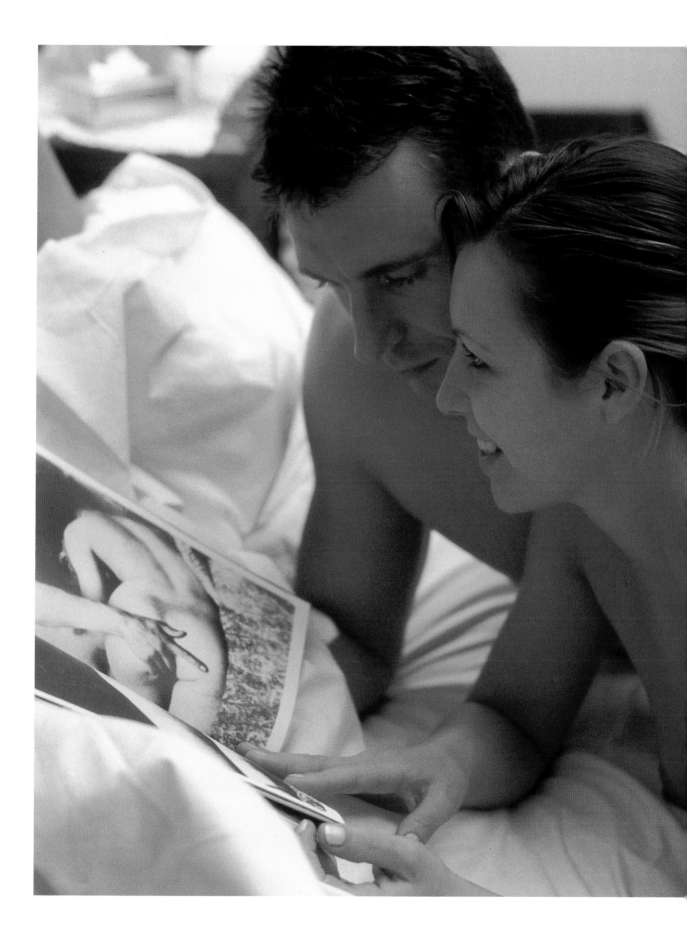

Tantric bliss

The art of tantric sex can take years to perfect – but you can introduce some tantric techniques into your sex life to add variety and help sex last longer. Yogis who traditionally practised tantra believed that a man wasted vital energy in ejaculating, so they developed ways of holding off ejaculation. At the same time they encouraged women to have as many orgasms as they could, in the belief that female sexuality was not just a pleasure in itself, but the source of all life energy.

Trying it out

The ultimate tantric experience for a man is to learn how to have orgasms without ejaculating, so that his penis can stay hard for hours, with orgasm after orgasm. Experts use yoga and meditation in tantric sex. But for a beginner, the key points to remember are to take your time, to practise holding a pose instead of thrusting, and to maintain eye contact with your partner – something that's probably much more difficult than you think.

Start with the man sitting on the floor and his partner sitting astride him in his lap. Instead of her bouncing up and down, just hold one another, occasionally rocking back and forth. Gaze into each other's left eye... What happens? See how long you can keep this up.

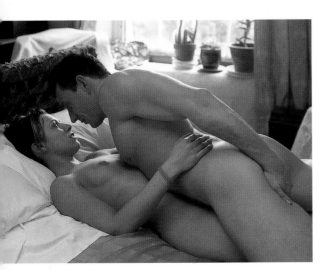

Tantric techniques for lasting longer

Stop thrusting. Stay still and take deep, regular breaths, breathing from your belly not your chest. Concentrate on your breathing until the urgency has passed.

Stay completely still, relax the genital and anal muscles and press your tongue against the roof of your mouth behind your teeth. Concentrate on the contact your tongue is making until your erection subsides sufficiently.

Withdraw your penis a little, so only the glans remains inside the vagina. Hold the position until the urgency has passed, then slowly enter the vagina again.

Vary your strokes so that you don't get carried away by the rhythm and hurtle towards climax.

Press your index finger and thumb on your perineum, midway between the anus and scrotum. Keep up the pressure until your erection has subsided slightly.

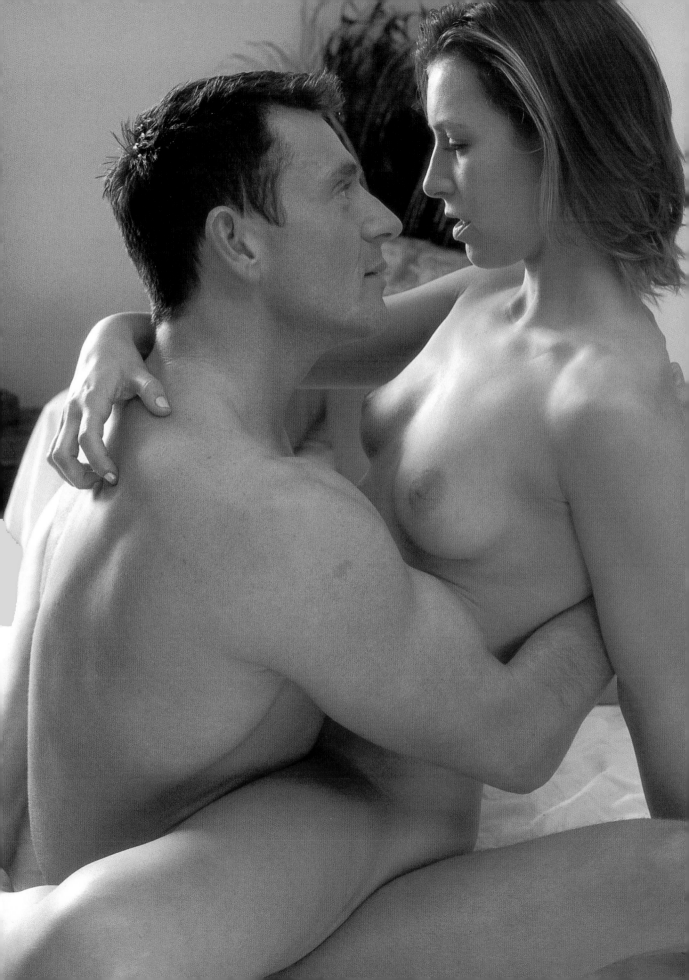

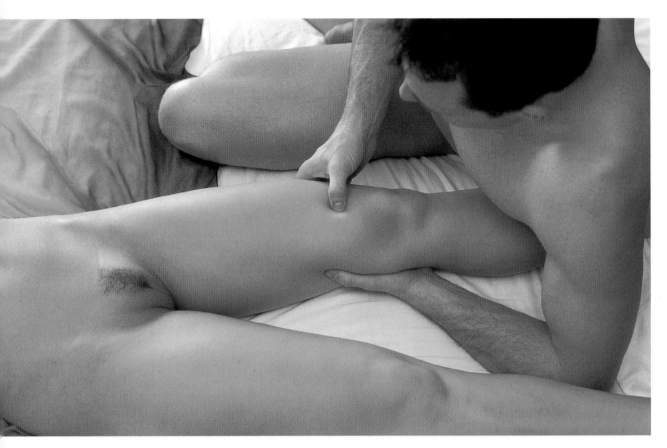

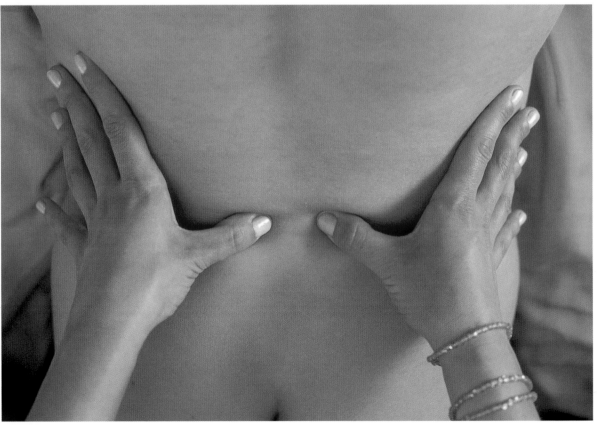

Pressure boost

Try a regular massage of specific pressure points to boost your sexual energy. The Japanese therapy of shiatsu is based on the philosophy and medical theory of acupuncture. It means 'finger pressure', but therapists also use the palms of their hands and sometimes elbows, knees and feet to apply stronger pressure. Shiatsu works with the flow of energy called ki that runs through the body in channels known as meridians. By working pressure points along these meridians, blockages can be dissolved and the flow of energy released.

The kidney meridian

Sexuality is governed by the kidney meridian. The kidney pressure points, or *tsubos*, are found about one thumb's width, or *cun*, on either side of the spine, level with the space between the second and third lumbar vertebrae. Work both left and right *tsubos* at once.

You know when you have found the *tsubo* when your thumb nestles into a small hollow. If it feels full of energy, with strong muscle tone or a sharp tender feeling, keep your thumb on the spot, or make small circling or pumping motions until you feel the energy relax. If energy is lacking and the *tsubo* feels empty and needy, hold your thumb in the spot until you feel the energy return.

It takes years to train as a professional shiatsu practitioner, but here are some pressure points that you can experiment with on your partner at home – work them to increase and strengthen the flow of their sexual energy.

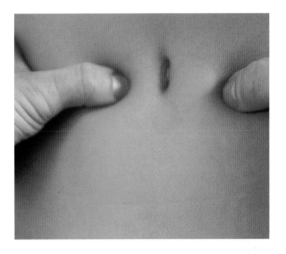

Acupressure points for good sex

Meeting Point of the Three Yin Leg Meridians – 3 *cun* (thumb's widths) above the tip of the ankle bone, push into the edge of the tibia. Especially useful when periods are irregular.

Heavenly Pivot – 2 *cun* either side of the navel. Good for relieving menstrual pain.

Ocean of Blood – 3 *cun* above the kneecap on the bulge of the muscle. As the name indicates, this is also good for menstrual pain.

Kidney Back Transporting Point – 1.5 *cun* to the sides of the spine, level with the space between the second and third lumbar vertebrae. Excellent for lack of sexual desire in either sex.

Greater Stream – right between the ankle bone and the Achilles tendon. Treats lack of vitality and sexual energy.

Gate of Life – between the second and third lumbar vertebrae. Boosts vitality and libido.

Gate to Original Ki – 3 *cun* below the navel – good for fatigue and boosting the libido.

Sexercise

Sex is the best exercise ever – and exercise and fitness make for better sex. Keeping in good shape means you have more energy, alertness, confidence and stamina – you look and feel more attractive. With an improved self-body image, you'll never be embarrassed by nakedness. Added benefits for men who get rid of their gut are that more sex positions become accessible – and a leaner body makes the penis look and feel bigger because it's no longer shrouded in fat. Exercise raises the blood levels of hormones involved in the chemistry of arousal – it makes you want sex more urgently, more often. So why not exercise together?

Work out then make out

Spend one hour every other day doing vigorous aerobic exercises. In one study, 50-year-old male office workers with erection problems did this for nine months – by which time they were making love 30 per cent more often than they had been when they started. A control group walked for one hour every other day – with no recorded benefits to their sex lives.

If you have an exercise bench, use it for robust sexercises in which you thrust against one another. She lies on her back and pushes by holding on to support bars, while he stands between her legs.

Go running together, pacing yourselves well against each other, take a hot shower together afterwards, then fall on each other and make love, invigorated.

Dancing is terrific exercise. The invention of ballroom dancing scandalized polite society because it involved erotic clinching in public. Now we don't need an excuse to embrace, dancing has become more energetic and fluid, so put all your powers of seduction into the way you move. Combine it with stripping, or undress each other. Try carrying positions for making love to music. Prefer something more structured? Take classes in salsa, or learn the tango, the sexiest dance on Earth.

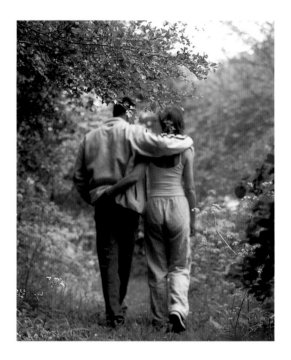

Play a hard game of tennis, badminton, or squash – the competitive element is a great turn-on.

Ego boost. Show off by working out at a gym – a good place to meet other people in training to build sexy bodies. Lots of people get turned on by seeing each other work up a sweat. Most gyms offer a personal programme of exercises tailored to your needs and abilities.

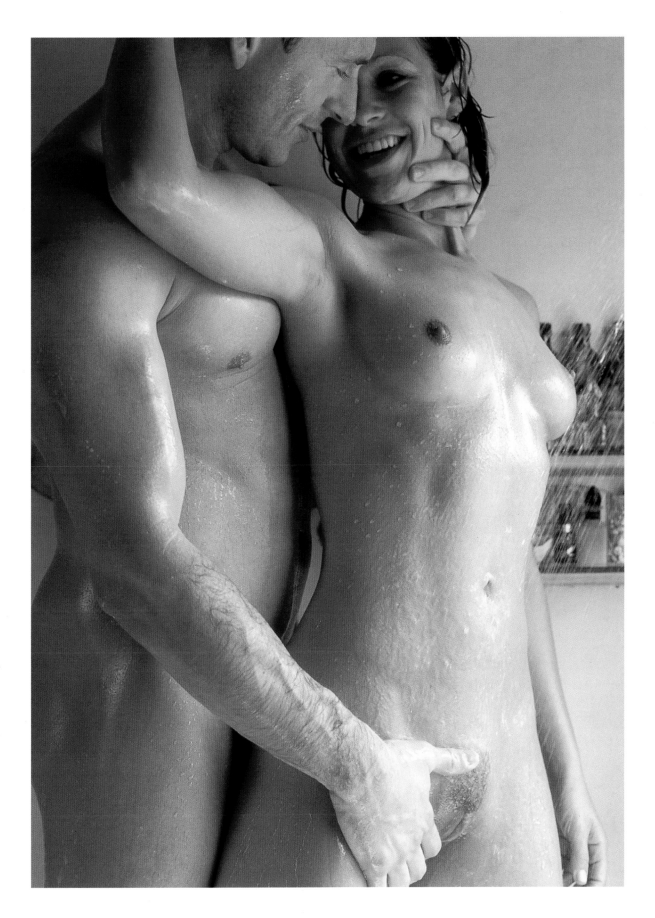

Condoms

Goat bladders, sheep intestines, linen bags – all have been used in the past to make a sheath for the penis in the hope of preventing pregnancy. Casanova used half a lemon. Condoms have come a long way since then, however. Today's best are made of ultra-thin latex and are far more pleasant to use.

Safe and sexy

Condoms are 88 per cent safe. They offer the only method of protection against sexually transmitted diseases, so if you're uncommitted, restless and sexually adventurous or just starting a new relationship, below are a few tips about how to make using a condom fun and sexy.

Latex or polyurethane?

Latex condoms need to be used with water-based lubricants such as KY jelly, as oil can damage the latex. Some people are allergic to latex – and they should try condoms made of polyurethane. Stronger and more expensive, they are safe to use with any lubricant, including oils.

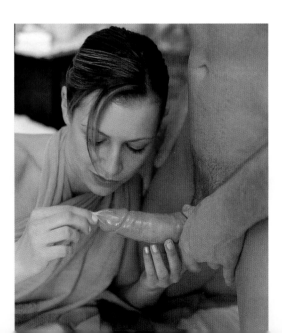

How to love latex

Go shopping for special condoms. Browse in sex shops or specialist catalogues, or surf the internet for something different. Try coloured or flavoured ones. Condoms with bobbles on them are designed to stimulate the vaginal walls and could help with finding her G-spot.

Breaking off from making love to put on a condom is likely to spoil the mood, so let your lover put it on for you. She first massages a drop of lubricant on to the tip of your penis with her finger, then squeezes the teat at the tip of the condom to expel the air. She places the opening of the condom on the glans and unrolls it down the sheath to fit comfortably. She can use her lips as well as her fingers to smooth it snugly along the shaft – some women claim to be able to put on a condom using their mouths alone.

Water-based lubricants tend not to last very long and need re-applying. Use saliva, or keep a small plant mister by the bed and add the delicate sensation of the spray to your lovemaking menu.

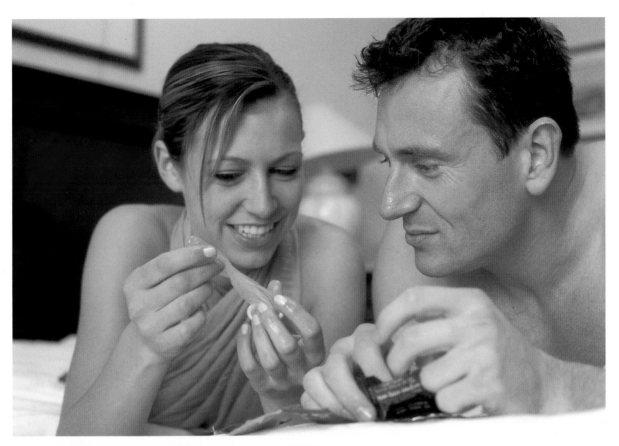

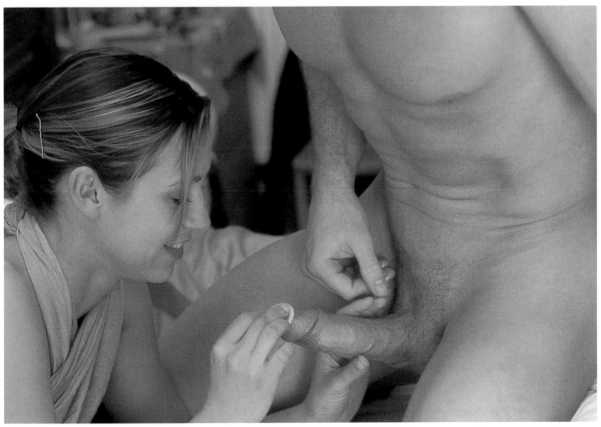

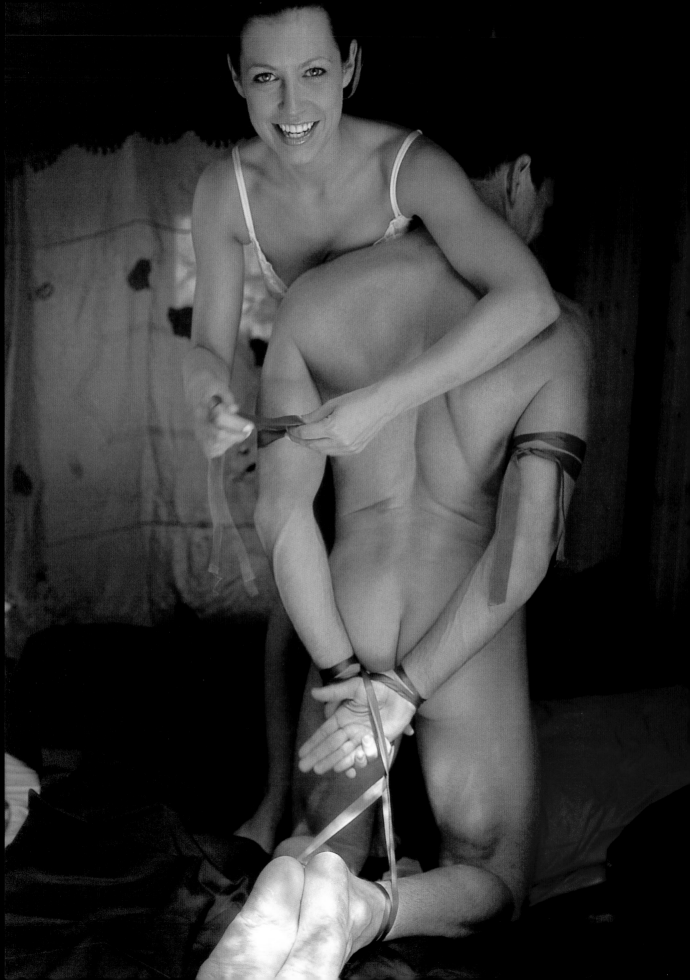

TOY BOX

Planning erotic games ahead increases the anticipation and excitement. So every few weeks, make a date with your lover when you'll have more than a couple of hours to spare and devote it to trying something new – take it in turns to choose what will be on the sexual menu. The preparation – finding a video that's both explicit enough for him and erotic enough for her, buying underwear that will drive him wild, adding edible body paints to your toy box and fixing up a swing in the bedroom – these should all be part of the thrill.

Lingerie

Beautiful underwear boosts a woman's self-confidence – and a man's morale – only he will get to know what she wears under her clothes when they're out together. Perhaps it's a filmy teddy, a lacy bustier, or stockings and suspenders... with nothing else. Lingerie makes a woman feel pampered and luxurious, it belongs in the same seductive part of the imagination as high heels and make-up – and in the bedroom it allows her to play the vamp.

The buyer's guide

Men who buy women sexy underwear are sometimes accused of buying themselves a present – put this right by taking your partner along to choose the gift herself. She's the expert on fit, style and the colour to suit her skin, she knows whether she wants lace or leopard. Most importantly, she knows what makes her feel sexy – and if it's magic for her it will work for you too. And in the shop you'll get to see her model a whole selection of gorgeous lingerie.

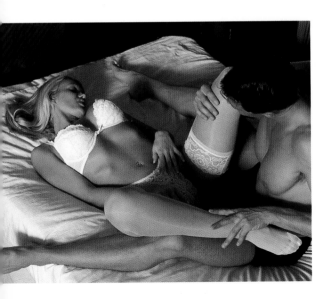

A man's guide to women's underwear

A woman can use lingerie to send a signal her partner won't miss – dressing for bed in a cosy nightie and a pair of woolly socks means she needs a good night's sleep, but appearing in a black lace bustier means something else...

A teddy is an all-in-one with a fitted bra top – go for filmy, lacy Lycra.

A camisole is a fitted top that sometimes incorporates a bra. They come in soft cotton knits or fresh crisp broderie anglaise, which is a cotton fabric decorated with little embroidered holes.

The craze for corsets has revived with the bustier, a sexy one-piece sculptured garment that incorporates an uplift-bra, nips in at the waist and hugs her figure as far as the hips. This very dressy item comes in luxury fabrics and finishes and luscious colours. The right fit will do wonders for almost every figure – so make this your choice for a special gift, but let her try it first.

A suspender belt and stockings is something you can buy as a surprise – you'll need to know her waist, hip and shoe size.

Something else you can safely buy her if you know her size is a selection of silk bikini thongs. At the front is the merest scrap of colour and at the back, a thong that disappears between her buttocks. A thong is great for emphasizing a curvaceous behind and is invisible under even the thinnest pair of trousers.

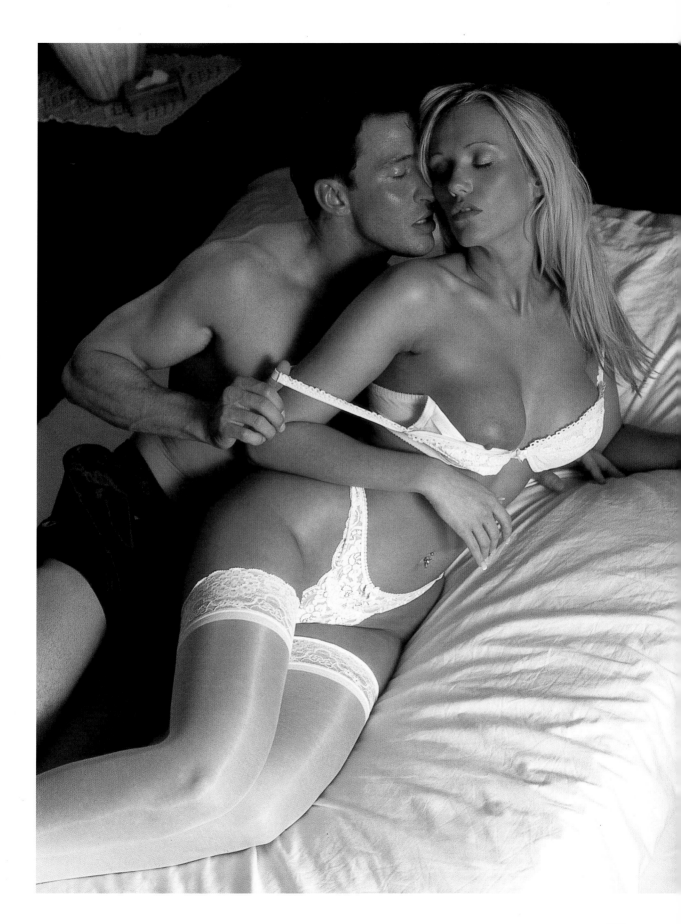

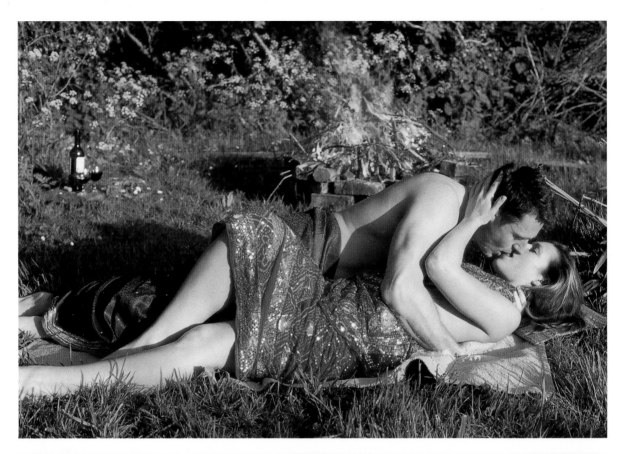

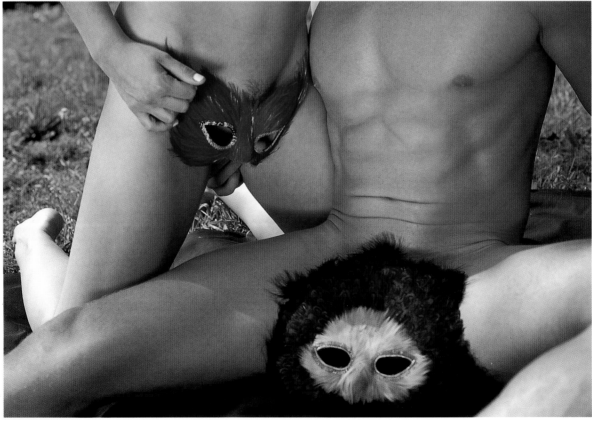

Sex god

Does your lover have a secret longing to be a glamorous rock-star? Would you like to play groupie to an androgynous god? Exploring the characteristics of the opposite sex within ourselves is an intriguing part of understanding the human psyche. In the interests of breaking down the boundaries of sexism – while treating yourself to a powerful erotic turn-on – vamp up your man to give him a mysteriously ambivalent new sexuality.

Turning the tables

Women can express their feelings about power and domination by wearing masculine clothes any day of the week, but it's a different matter for men – Western dress codes deny them a whole world of colour and sensuousness. So lock the door, get out the make-up and get imaginative. Act out your fantasy. Think of Queen Zinua of Angola. In the 17th century she was famous for keeping a whole collection of husbands permanently dressed as women. You needn't go quite that far, however.

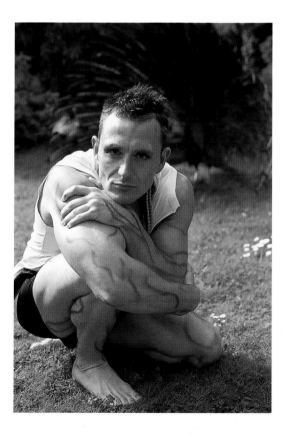

Pamper your partner

Relax him first with a proper beauty session. Give him a luxurious bath and shampoo with scalp massage followed by an all-over body rub with aromatherapy oils and a facial. Put cucumber slices on his eyelids, play music, work magic on his skin with dreamy fingers.

Apply just a touch of make-up – darken his lashes with mascara and add mystery to his eyes with kohl. Subtly redden his lips. If he is dark-skinned, add lustrous highlights and a touch of gold or bronze blusher. Manicure and buff his nails or add pearly varnish that tones with his skin. Turn him into a film star.

Now experiment with clothes – think drama, glamour, beauty – and create an appearance that you both love to look at. Try torn T-shirts, jewels, a studded leather collar, or the thrilling contrast of a delicate fabric like silk against a rough male skin.

The perfect way to end this particular game is for the newly created sex god to act out a fantasy. Let him take charge and make love to him in any way he wants to.

Body painting

In ancient societies and ethnic tribes, body painting was and is a ritual art form. Before hunting or warfare, people use natural pigments and the juices of plants to decorate themselves to look like wild animals or sacred spirits. In sex play, body painting can be used like a mask to release inhibitions and set a mood. It can inspire erotic dancing, or it can be enjoyed just for itself – beautifying the body of your beloved to music is an absorbing act of love.

Choosing your paint

In India, a bride's hands and feet are often decorated with intricate patterns painted in henna, a process that may take several days to complete and is an important part of preparation for the marriage bed. You can buy henna in packets with instructions for painting and templates for hand and foot patterns inside. Henna stains the skin dark red-brown for a few days.

You can also try customized body paints. Some are flavoured and designed to be licked off afterwards. Read the label to check whether they will stain the sheets.

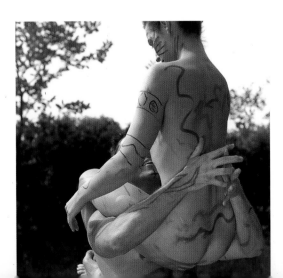

Body art

Select the location and music to match your mood and the design you are about to create.

Begin by giving your partner a full body massage with oil to seal dry, porous skin.

With your lover standing, apply the paints with a large soft brush, following the contours of the body. Use dramatic flowing strokes, working delicately around particularly sensitive areas such as breasts, palms, face and genitals. Make it a truly sensual experience.

Add a dusting of glitter or work body transfers into your design. You could use transfers of birds and flowers to create a tropical rainforest.

Paint each other and dance together against a suitable backdrop. Take photographs of yourselves.

As you make love, the colours merge and spread. Take another photograph afterwards before you wash it all off.

Caution Test paints on a small patch of skin first and don't use if there is an allergic reaction. Remember the film *Goldfinger*! Don't completely cover the body in paints as sweat glands may be blocked, which stops the body from regulating its own temperature and can be dangerous.

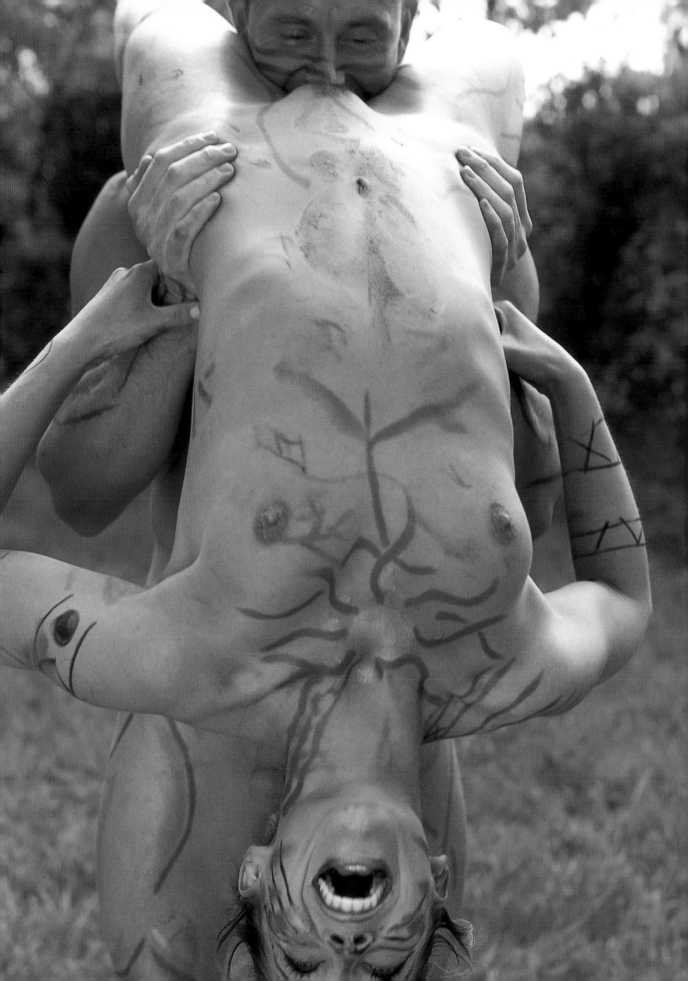

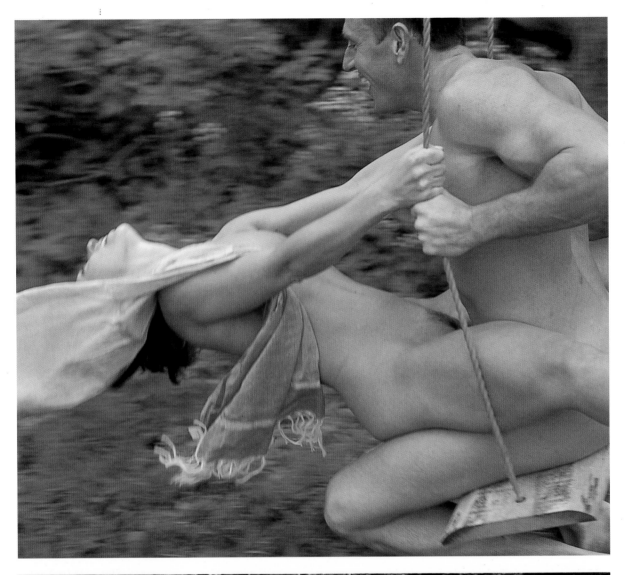

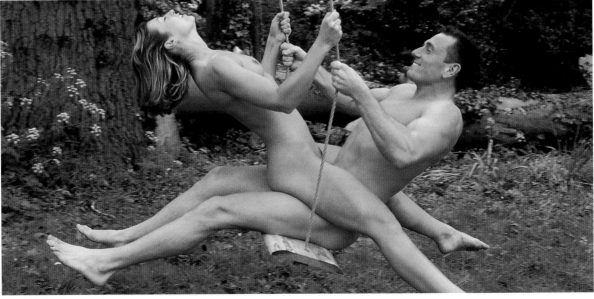

Swings

The *Kama Sutra* records that in the royal pleasure gardens of ancient India there were always swings for lovers hung in trees or among the fragrant blooms of shaded bowers. Using swings in lovemaking adds its own rhythm and gives a lovely sensation of being near to weightlessness. Swings also allow lovers to experiment with different angles and positions as they fly through the air – or bump heavily against one another.

Making a swing

If you don't have a suitable tree or a shaded bower in your garden, it should be easy enough to fix one up in your bedroom. The most crucial point is that the fixings should easily take both your weights and the momentum you generate, so you'll need a strong beam or joist on which to fix it. Take the swing down when not in use and hang lanterns on the hooks.

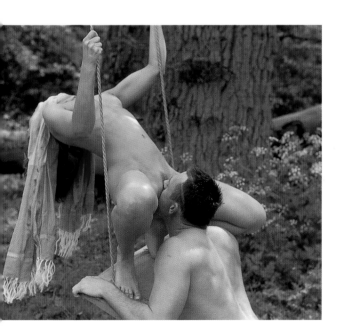

Things to do on swings

Tantalize, fantasize, to get in the mood. He lies on the bed, she swings towards him allowing her skirt to fly up in the breeze.

Cunnilingus. This is most comfortable on a trapeze swing. She holds on to the ropes of the swing and, remaining upright, lowers herself so the swing is under her bent knees. He kneels on the ground in front of her. In this position he can also push her very gently backwards and forwards.

Have several hooks on the ropes of your swing so that you can alter its height. Then you can go for cunnilingus with the man standing, or have her swinging at his hip height so that he can penetrate her from the front. He can precision-control her movement with his hands on her hips to create vigorous or exquisitely delicate sensations.

He sits on the swing, she sits on his lap, moving herself up and down with her hands on the ropes.

Two swings. Another idea from the *Kama Sutra*. Hang the swings about 30 cm (12 inches) apart so you will always move together. Sit on the swings facing one another with your legs around the outside of the ropes. A brilliant position for using your hands as well as penetration.

Basket swing. Remember those cocoon-shaped basket swings? Get one with a large hole in the seat and suspend it at the right height for cunnilingus. Disguise it with a board over the hole and a cushion on it when not in use.

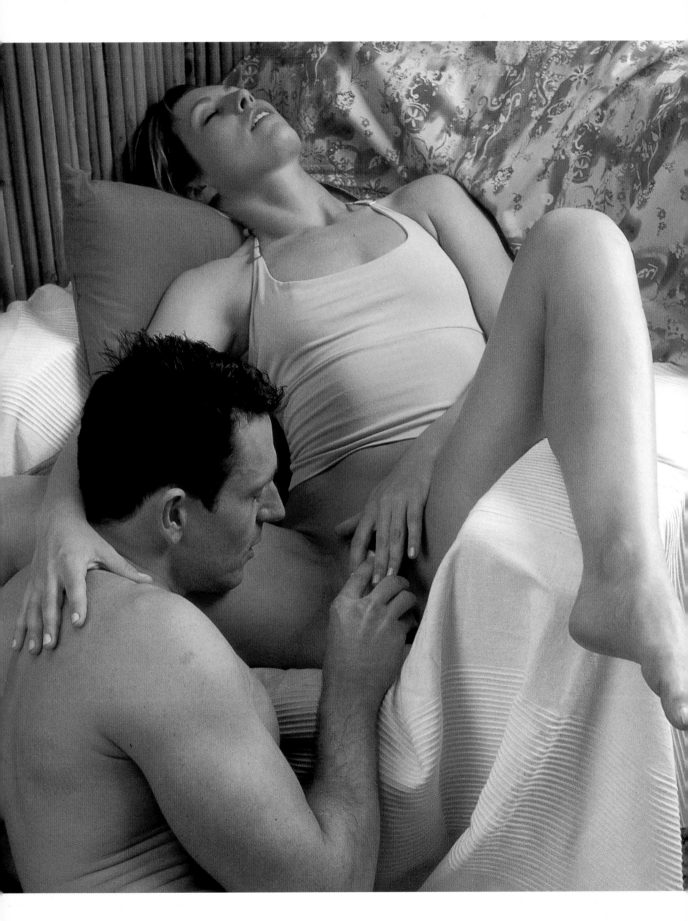

Vibrators

Dildos – even double dildos that could be used by two women – have been known since Stone Age times. Phallic toys were also popular in ancient Egypt and Greece, and Indian sultans gave them to the ladies of the harem in an attempt to keep them sexually satisfied and to discourage lesbianism.

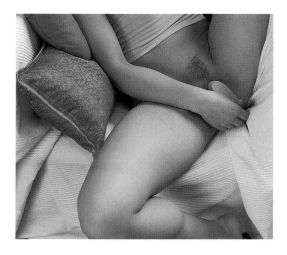

Good vibrations

The first electrical dildos, or vibrators, were produced in America around 1910. They were large cumbersome machines designed to be used by doctors on female patients suffering from hysteria – 'womb disease' – what we today would call sexual frustration. But it wasn't until the feminist revolution of the 1960s and 70s that women began to talk openly about the fact that orgasm is not always easily achieved through penetration, and vibrators started to be marketed as a sexual device.

Most vibrators today are phallus-shaped, many are made from skin-friendly materials such as silicon and Cyberskin, and some have computer chips and a 10-speed push-button remote control. The most reliable types plug into the mains, though the most convenient models are battery driven. The latest battery-operated vibrators, designed by a woman called Candida Royalle, are shaped like a curved mobile phone and fit snugly into the vulva. Their tremendous popularity signals that the days of the phallic vibrator may be numbered.

Vibrator hints and tips

A massage with a good vibrating massager is an excellent relaxant as a prelude to languid sex.

Always add plenty of lubricant when using a vibrator.

You can learn your partner's masturbation technique by watching her use her vibrator.

Some men like to have the tip of a vibrator inserted into the anus during fellatio.

Some women like a vibrator inserted into the vagina during cunnilingus, or use one to stimulate the clitoris while having sex facing away from and astride their partner.

Try pressing a small vibrator behind your tongue as you lick her clitoris with the tip of it.

Either put a fresh condom on your vibrator every time or wash it in a baby-bottle sterilizing solution after use and dry it before storing.

Some people don't like sex toys. Never try to persuade anyone to try one against their will.

Novelties

Let's start with lighting. Do you like to make love with the light on or off? Harsh light is unkind to lovers, so pay attention to the lighting in your bedroom. Choose pools of soft light away from the bed so that you can see enough to read each other's eyes. Try dusky pink, red or even black light bulbs, which are easy on the eyes and give pale skin a healthy glow. Alternatively, fit a dimmer switch that can be reached from the bed. Candlelight is the softest and most flattering of all, but make sure candles don't get knocked over and remember to blow them out before you fall asleep.

Little extras

Music Some people find music distracting, others choose it to match their mood. Try swooning to Wagner's *Liebestod* or let your favourite band drive the pace.

Mask OK, you know very well who your partner is, but the anonymity of a glamorous mask can give an extra frisson of danger and strip away inhibitions you never knew you had.

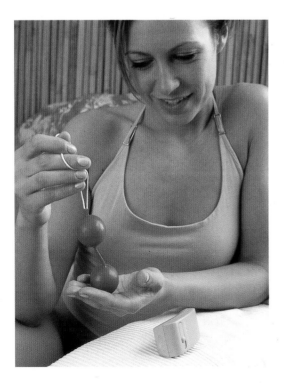

Rubber Some people just love the sensual feel of rubber – others hate it. Tight rubber clothes are best put on with a generous dusting of talcum powder to help them glide over the skin. Rubber gear is traditionally black and meant to get wet.

Ripping stuff Ever fancied ripping the clothes off your lover? Keep some of your old T-shirts specially for the purpose.

Penile ring Worn at the base of the penis, these rings are claimed by some men to stiffen the erection. Some have a knob on the upper side designed to stimulate the clitoris. A tape runs through the ring, over the scrotum and anus, and attaches to a tape around the waist.

Caution: rings that are too tight sometimes have to be removed in hospital.

Blakoe ring This encircles the base of the penis and scrotum and is worn to produce a pleasant sensation of tightness. In China and Japan, professionals bind the base of the penis with strips of leather to produce the same result.

Caution: Beware of cutting off the blood supply or bruising the urethra.

Chinese balls or eggs A pair of egg-shaped balls designed to be put in the vagina and worn all day. The balls are hollow, usually made of plastic, and have smaller, solid metal balls inside them that create a strange sensation as the woman moves.

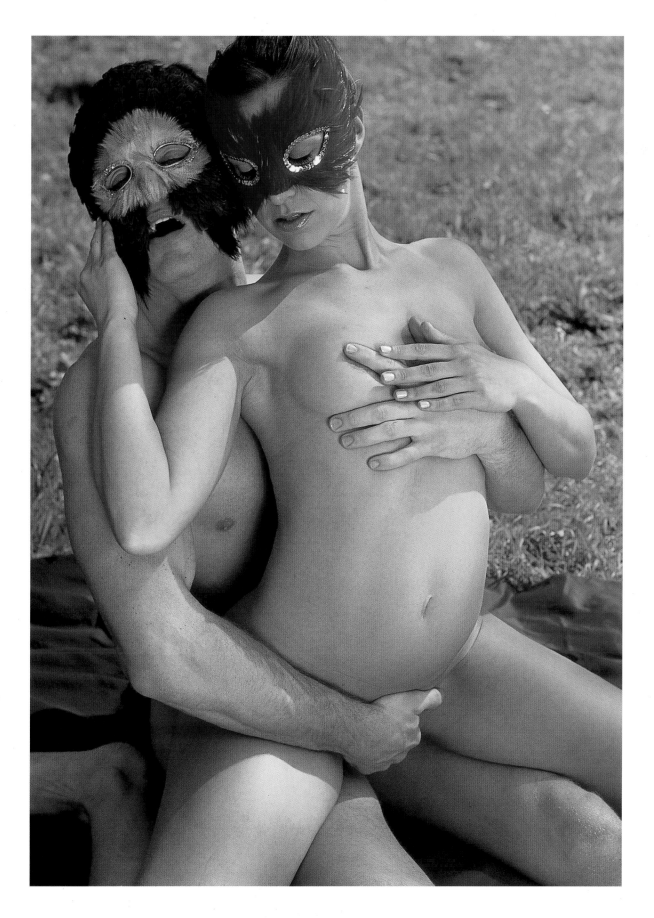

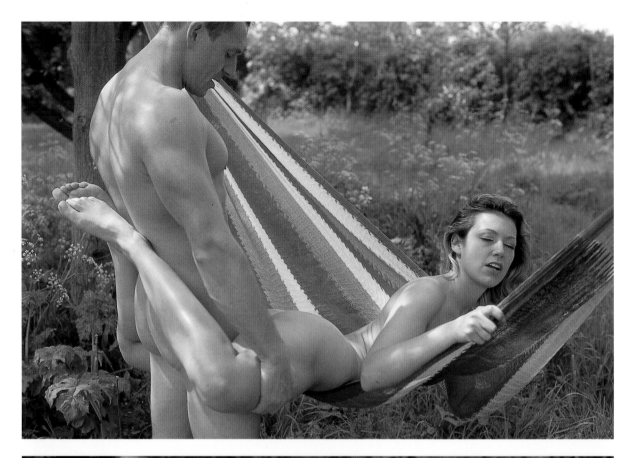

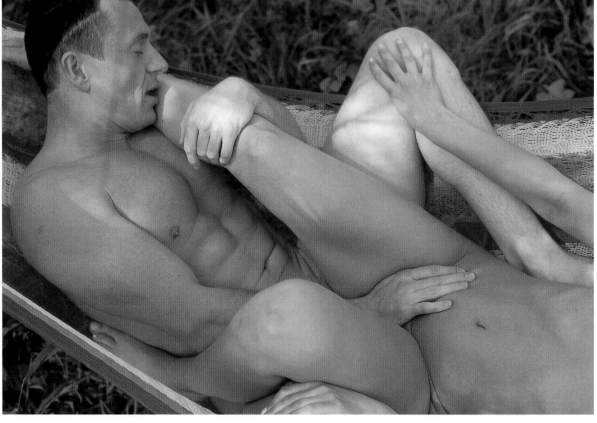

Hammock

Hang a double hammock in your garden or in the bedroom, making sure the fixings are strong enough to take the two of you plus some energetic movement. A hammock provides a wonderful private cocoon in which to make love, and afterwards its gentle movement can lull you to sleep in one another's arms. A great way to spend a Sunday afternoon. The lazy curve of the hammock means that some flat-out positions, such as the missionary, are ruled out. Here are a few alternatives to try.

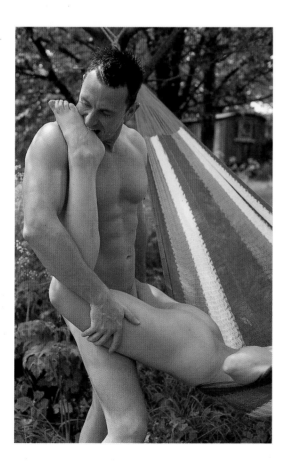

How to make love in a hammock

Side-by-side. He lies facing her back and enters from behind. Also called the spoons position because of the neat way the two bodies fit together.

Soixante-neuf side-by-side. Discover that a hammock is the ideal environment for long lazy mutual oral sex.

The lovers lie on their sides facing each other. She lifts her upper leg over his body and he enters her underneath it. These side-by-side positions are good for gently swinging in the hammock.

He lies on his back, for comfort dangling his legs over the sides of the hammock from his knees. She sits astride him with her legs outside the hammock, supporting her hands on his shoulders as she moves up and down.

Use the hammock as a swing. She lies face down across the hammock, her legs hanging towards the ground. He kneels in front of her to give her oral sex, then stands up to penetrate her from behind, using the swinging movement of the hammock to help him thrust against her.

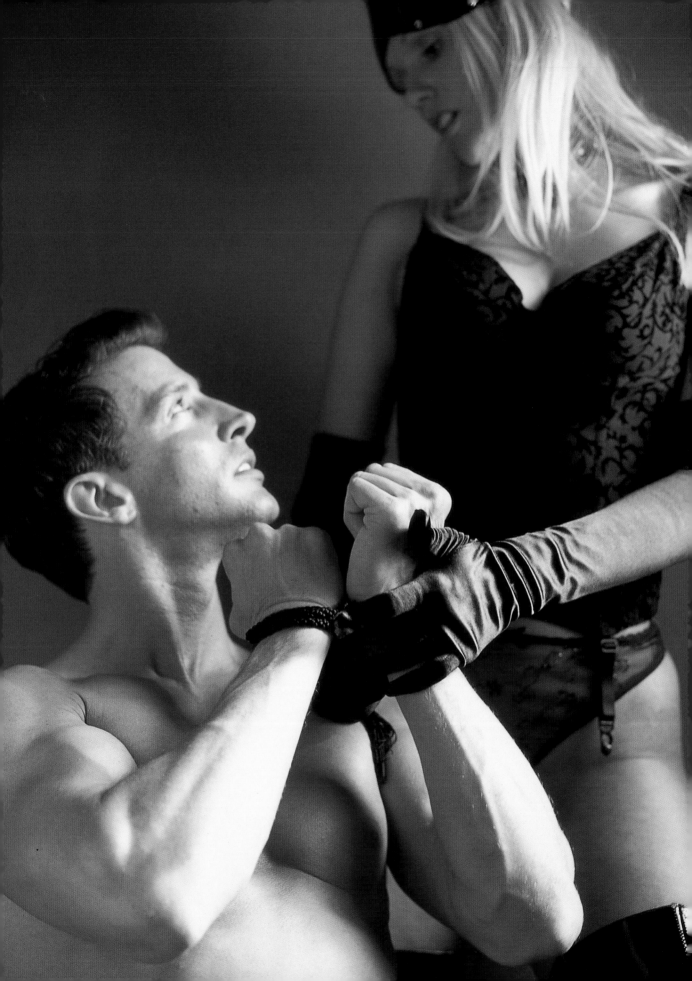

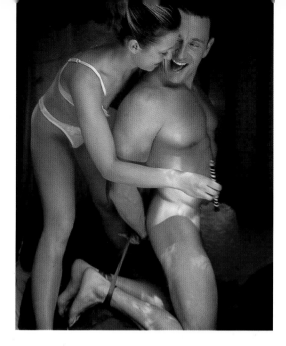

Bondage

The thought of bondage and dominance in a loving relationship may sound weird, but for some couples it's merely a harmless and exciting way of exploring feelings they're denied in everyday life. The idea is to enhance your sex life and discover more about each other through play acting – it's not a licence for cruelty. The dominant partner – the 'top' is in charge of ensuring that the submissive partner, or 'bottom', has a good time and doesn't get hurt.

No pressure

What's in it for the top? He or she gets to do anything they like, and can have anything they like done to them. For the bottom, it's a chance to relinquish responsibility for the sex act and explore aspects of sexuality that they might otherwise be too shy or embarrassed to try. It's also liberating in that it completely eliminates performance anxiety.

Try these fantasies

- Cleopatra and her slave
- Empress Catherine the Great and a soldier in her army
- Sultan and harem

Try these techniques

- Tickling with a feather, tassel or silk scarf
- Temptation with dance, strip-tease and story-telling
- Long languid oral sex

Before you tie up your partner

Always discuss what you are going to do and how long it will last. Never tie anyone up against their will.

Use safe ties. Don't do anything that will cut off air supply or circulation. Don't use slip knots, as they tighten when pulled. Comfortable furry handcuffs are sold at sex shops. Keep the handcuff key nearby, or have a pair of scissors handy in case you need to loosen ties quickly.

Don't leave anyone alone once you have bound them up.

Since shouting: 'No! no! no!' might well be part of your game, agree on an escape word before you start – and end the game immediately you hear it. Some couples use 'yellow' and 'red' to slow and stop the game, or you might prefer a non-verbal signal, such as clicking the fingers.

Don't play this game when under the influence of drink or drugs.

Avoid expressing or arousing real anger and aggression during the game.

Sex on film

It used to be assumed that women weren't turned on by sex on celluloid – until therapist Patricia Love conducted laboratory experiments that proved the opposite. In fact one US survey says that 40 per cent of soft porn video rentals are taken out by women. However, it's unfortunately true that most films featuring explicit sex are made by men for men – with masturbation in mind.

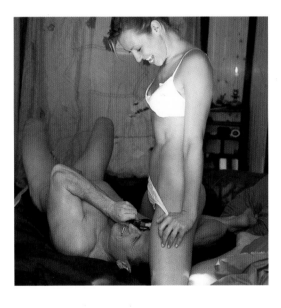

Explicit porn

Most porn films come short on preliminaries, characterization and plot, they focus almost entirely on what goes on between two or more sets of genitals and feature serial anonymous sex sessions. Women might enjoy their partners' arousal but are likely to become bored and scathing about this unsophisticated form of cinema after watching two or three. Which is not what either of you wants. So here are a few ideas to help you find films that are erotic enough for her and explicit enough for him.

Erotic and explicit

Look for films made by Candida Royalle, who also invented the vulva-shaped vibrator. Her movies don't demean women or feature violent sex. They focus on female pleasure – so are a real turn-on for men too. Titles include *Christine's Secret*, *A Taste of Ambrosia* and *Cabin Fever*.

A film maker recommended by *Men's Health Magazine* is Andrew Blake. He produces movies that don't look as though they were made in someone's shed. He concentrates on glamour and luxury – the glossy magazine feel with sex thrown in. Try *House of Dreams*, *Femmes Erotiques* or *Hidden Obsessions*.

Be less deliberate about the whole thing – hire a mainstream video that just happens to feature steamy sex scenes and see where it takes you. Favourites are *Last Tango in Paris*, *Fatal Attraction* and *Basic Instinct*.

Be more deliberate about the whole thing – make your own erotic videos, setting up a camcorder in your bedroom – but never do this without your partner's full consent. Watching yourselves making love afterwards can be an eye-opener that breaks down inhibitions and gets your talking about which bits you liked best and what you might try next. You could concentrate on new techniques and positions or introduce costumes and fantasy storylines.

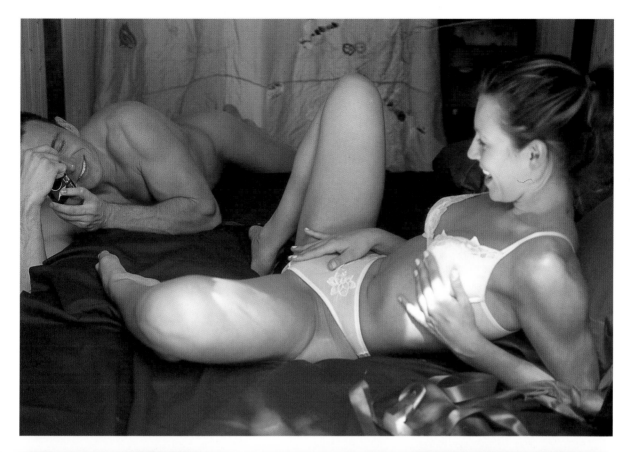

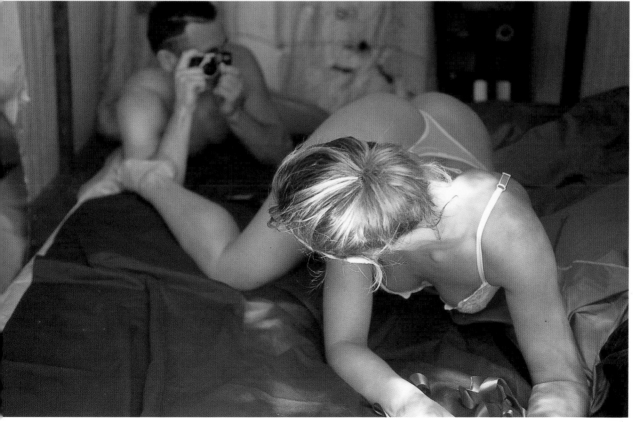

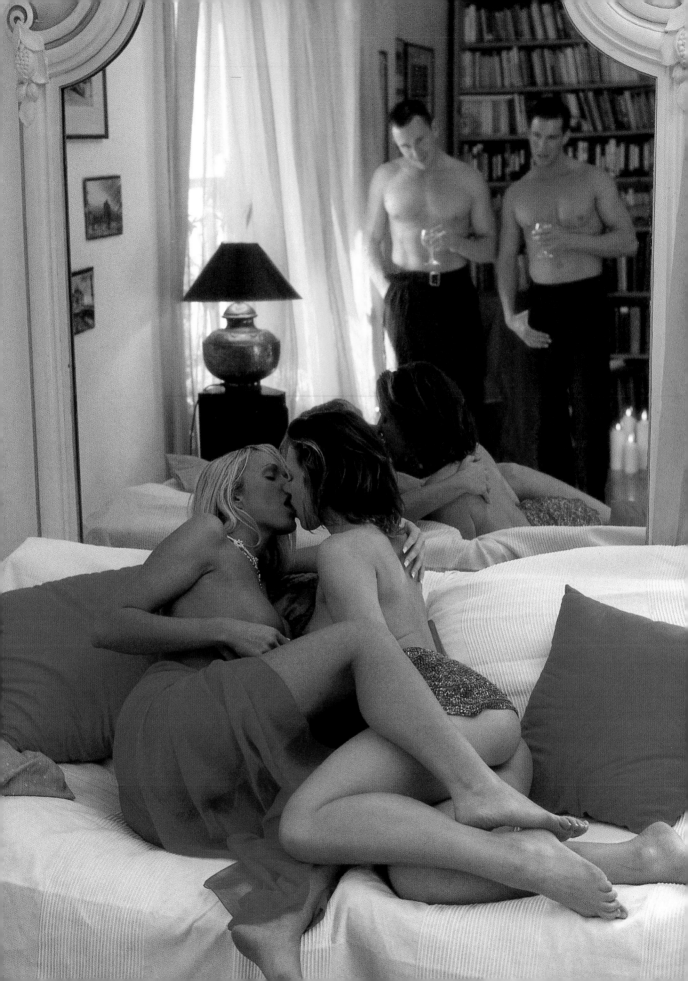

IN YOUR DREAMS

According to one survey 92 per cent of men and 87 per cent of women have fantasized about group sex, but only 13 per cent of men and 8 per cent of women admit to having tried it. Most prefer to stick to fantasy because that way they stay in control. The real thing involves the risk of complications. Don't do it to spice up a flagging sex life – it's more likely to deepen the rift between you. If you do experiment, discuss each other's motives fully first and think ahead to afterwards. Always practise safe sex and remember that oral-genital contact can transmit the HIV virus. In the meantime, carry on dreaming...

Mouth treats

Delicious food is a wonderful aphrodisiac, so serve it in the most sensual way you can imagine. Plan a naked picnic – or a picturesque lunch where some are naked and others are not. Throw a Roman banquet with musicians and bare-breasted dancers or an outdoor revel at the summer solstice... Feed each other with your lips and drink from each other's skin.

Erotic and delicious

In the pleasure quarters of Japan, men are often entertained to an erotic meal of sushi – tiny artistically presented parcels of fish, rice and vegetables – laid out on a human table – the body of a beautiful woman. Try it: the food is to be eaten without using the fingers – lips and tongues only!

Hors d'oeuvres to serve on a man's body: tiny pancake rolls, mini sausages, savoury rice rolled in fig leaves, a garland of vine leaves and grapes.

Hors d'oeuvres to serve on a woman's body – oysters and scallops in their shells, prawns arranged round a dip at the navel, baby artichokes, caviar.

Love noodles. Your naked male volunteer lies down and you place the plate over his genitals, drawing his penis and testicles through the hole. Pile the plate and his genitals with warm cooked spaghetti dressed in olive oil. Several of you sit around to eat. Drag the warm cooked spaghetti over his erection with your fingers, winding the strands around it and sucking them off.

Sweet anticipation

Nakedness tends to go well with foods that drizzle, squash, wobble or melt. Try chocolate, ice cream, extra virgin olive oil, raspberries, jelly, honey and molasses. Add edible flowers, such as nasturtiums. And don't forget that the way you eat can hold the promise of what you will do with your mouth and fingers later. Bear this in mind as you tear at the succulent flesh of a chicken leg or sink your teeth into a juicy ripe fig.

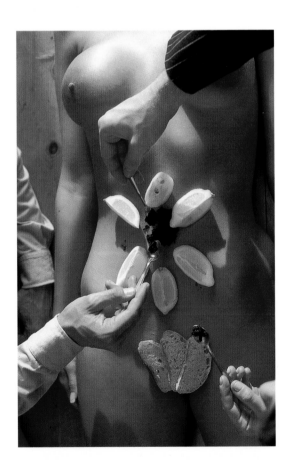

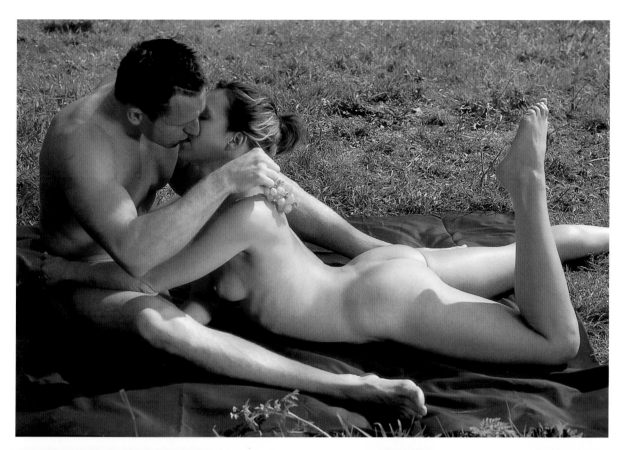

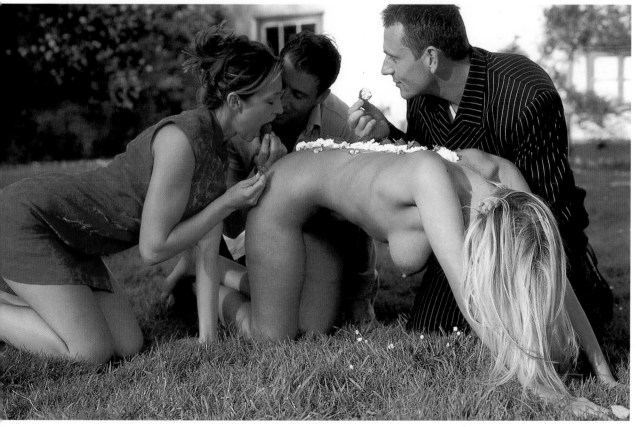

Playtime

Most of us probably started to learn about sex at an early age by playing games of doctors and nurses, and show and tell. Adult forays into new sexual territory can also mask hungry curiosity with riotous silliness – it shoos away the threat of taboo. So let your hair down and see what happens. Reintroduce playtime into your sex life and invent some games of your own. Start from here...

Daft things to do

Forfeits Saucy forfeits can be incorporated into any existing board game or card game, even table football. Have two sets of forfeits – one for parties and a more sensational one for just the two of you. Divide a small stack of blank cards between the players, who write their own forfeits on them· – anything from instructions to remove particular items of clothing, to commands such as 'lick the nipple of the person on your right 20 times'. Shuffle the cards, stack them up and start to play.

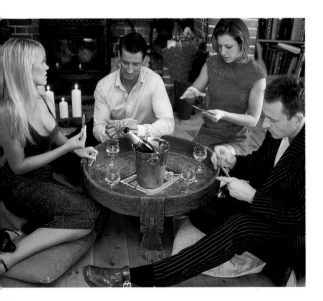

Another game of forfeits Have two sets of cards – one with actions, such as touch, tickle, kiss, suck, and another with body parts. The player has to follow the instructions, applying them to the correct body part.

And another in confessional mode There are incomplete sentences on the forfeit cards, such as, 'The first time I touched a naked man...'. The player has to complete the sentence.

Darts Write daft and sexy suggestions on pieces of paper pinned to a dart board. Then take it in turns throwing darts, and do whatever the speared pieces of paper tell you to.

Charades Each team gives the other the title of a blue movie or erotic book to enact. Imaginary titles are just as good as real ones.

When the music stops Play an adult version of this game, involving stripping or sexual favours.

Spin the bottle All stand in a circle and one player spins a bottle. The person the bottle ends up pointing at can request a sexual favour from anyone in the room.

Strip poker The winner of each hand gets to spend five minutes on their own with the person of their choice.

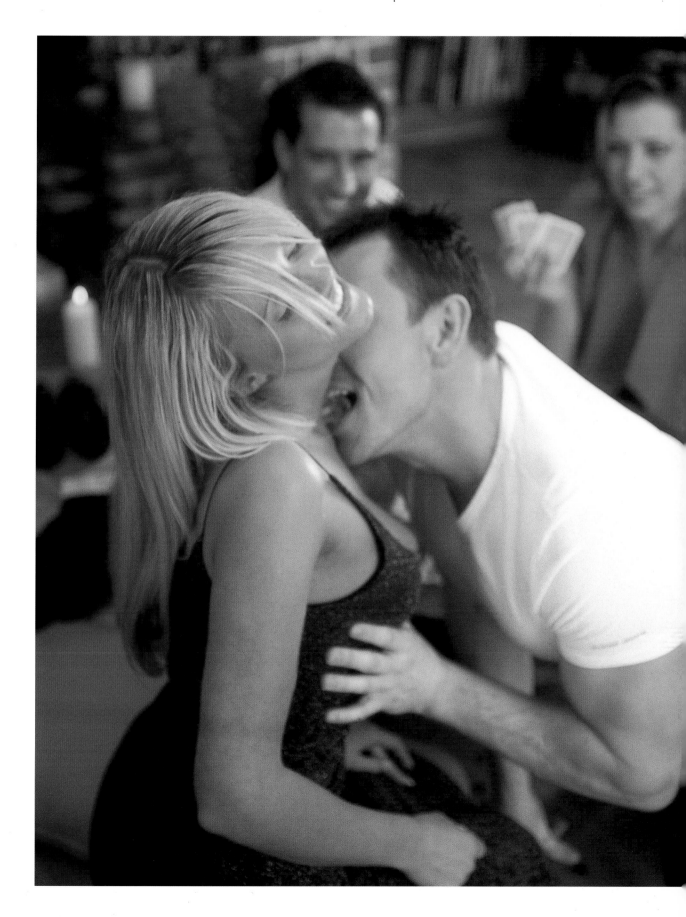

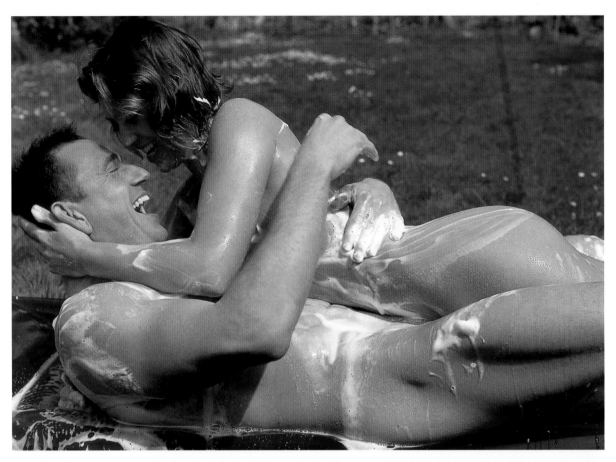

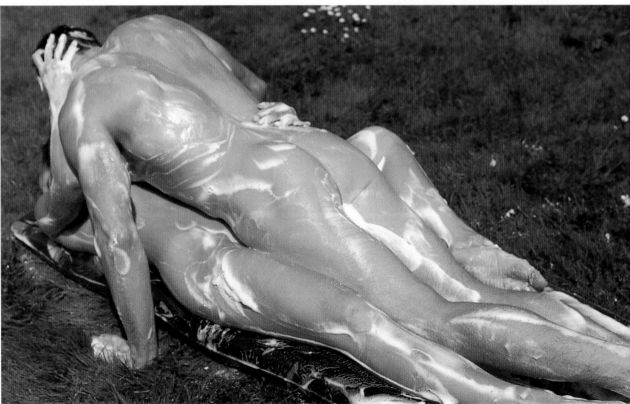

In a lather

Inunction is the seductive-sounding technical term for the act of rubbing someone with ointment or lather. During the carefree days of the 1960s when sex parties were at their peak in America, people would strip and rub lashings of cooking oil into each other's bodies, then find partners to slide against.

The joy of rubbing

If you use oil, choose almond oil for its light nutty smell, in preference to something usually used for frying chips. An alternative is warm soapy water. If the management will allow it, see if you can hire a local sauna for a party as the steamy atmosphere is good for the libido, and showers and plunge pools can be used for hot sex and cooling down.

If you want to give a lather party at home, provide futons covered with plastic sheets – which you can also lightly oil – plastic lilos, or best of all, a waterbed. Three of you can lie on the waterbed together, wriggling and writhing all over each other – to music, if you like. The slithery feeling is hot and quick, quite unlike the sensation of dry skin against dry skin. Set the rules beforehand – such as 'no hands' or 'no penetration'. In the bath houses of Bangkok, a handcuffed lathered man lies between two lathered women, also handcuffed, who writhe against him.

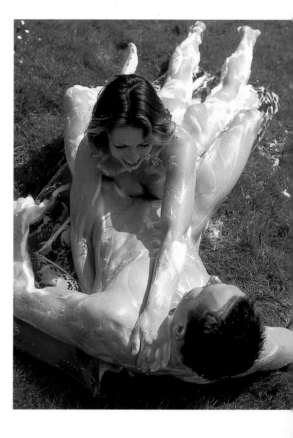

Lathering up

Try applying a soapy lather or sensuous oil on a rubber mitten with a nubbled palm for extra sensation.

Get your chosen partner to lie on a lilo and give him or her a bed bath with a hot flannel mitten, exploring and massaging the body in a thorough and leisurely fashion.

Cover an erect penis or open vulva with a fine silk scarf and drip oil on to it then massage with the palm, fingers and tongue – a lovely way to bring your partner to orgasm. Or do the same through silk underwear.

The X-zones

These games focus on the X-rated erogenous zones – the genitals and breasts. In the French erotic novel *The History of O* by the mysterious Pauline Réage, captives in the castle of love were instructed by their master never to wear clothing that would restrict sexual access. So the women wore fitted corsets tight enough to take their breath away but that left their breasts exposed and long skirts that were slashed up the front and gathered to the sides, revealing fishnet stockings and suspenders – and decoratively trimmed pubic hair. The men wore floor-length cloaks over black bodysuits, which had a hole cut in the front to expose their genitals.

X-zone outfits

Make yourselves some outfits like the ones in *The History of O* or have both sexes in body-hugging Lycra with strategically cut holes. Black blanks out the rest of the body, highlighting genitals and breasts to mesmerizing effect – especially if you also wear masks.

Topless

Topless fashions date from ancient Egypt and the Minoan civilization on Crete. Make yourself a topless dress with cleverly tied scarves, or cut up an old one. Surprise your partner by appearing in a familiar outfit - keep your back to him until you know you've got his attention, then turn round to reveal your new design!

Bottomless

This is one to play when you're in public. When no one else is looking, find a way of showing your partner that you've come out without your knickers. This is a good way of getting him to stay close to you all evening, with a protective hand caressing your bottom.

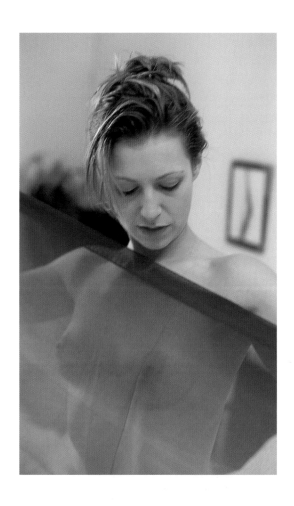

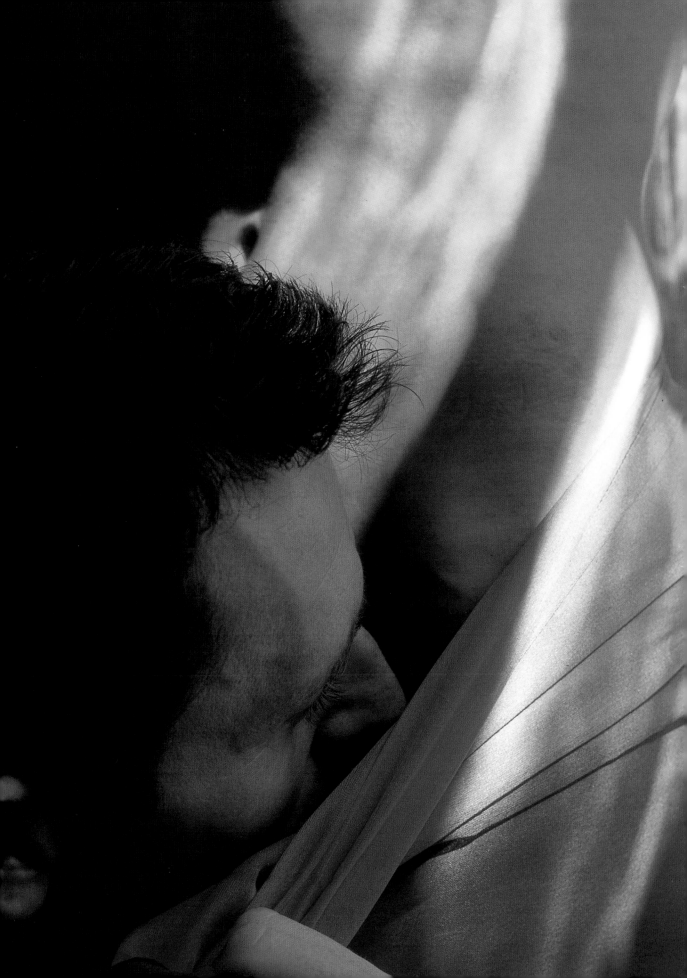

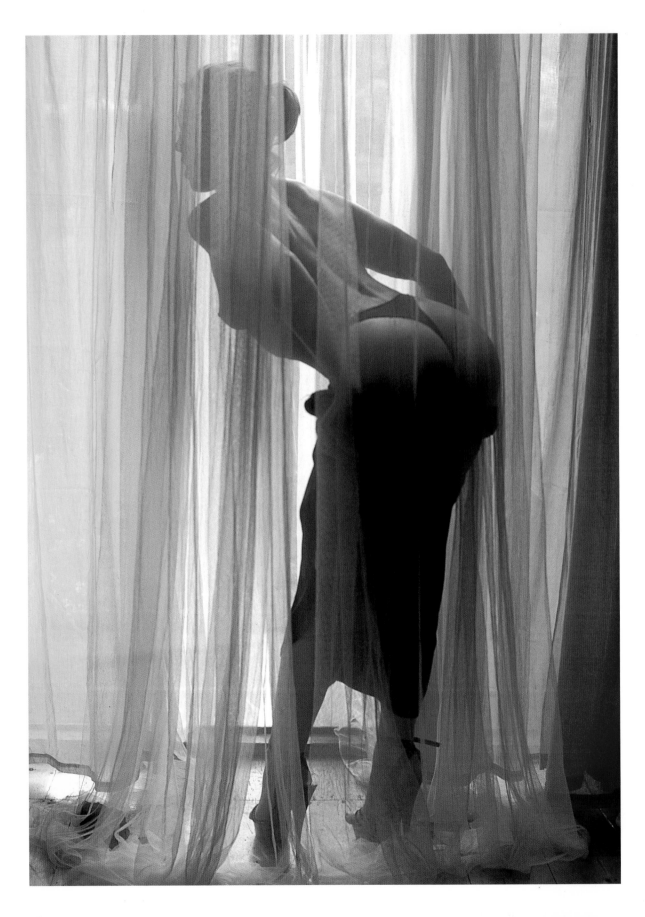

Silhouettes

The sight of two people illuminated as they make love behind a filmy curtain is unfailingly erotic. Veiled and yet revealed, the mystery and intimacy of sex is preserved as you watch, stirring the imagination and quickening the pulse. You can choose to play this game as a tease or do it for real.

Behind the veil

Suspend a wide gauzy curtain – it could be made of muslin or silk, or try a translucent shower curtain – from the ceiling in front of a lighted area, but keep the rest of the room where the audience sits dark. For a night-time garden party, the lovers can perform behind a muslin curtain hung at a lighted window and be watched from cushions on the lawn.

Couples volunteer in turns to perform behind the veil. They can't, of course, see their audience, so they are free to be as uninhibited and explicit as possible in their movements and gestures so that their silhouettes are clear. Any erotic acts are permitted whether simulated or for real – caressing, kissing, mutual masturbation, oral sex and intercourse – the object being to reveal as much as possible without actually being seen. Another twist is to award points to each couple and in one version of the game the audience can make special requests.

Each performance can begin with a striptease to music or erotic dancing. Below are some positions that will create good silhouettes.

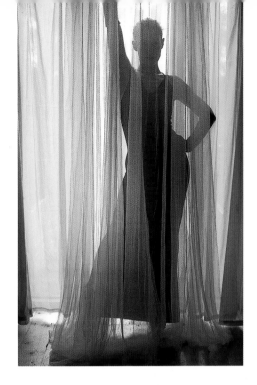

Six sex poses behind the veil

1. Fellatio – he stands sideways to the screen, she kneels in front of him.

2. Masturbation and mutual masturbation, sideways-on.

3. Cunnilingus – she stands sideways to the curtain, spreads her legs and leans over, supporting herself with her hands on a low stool. He kneels to lick her from behind.

4. From this position, he can stand and enter her from behind.

5. Wheelbarrow – she supports herself with her hands on the floor, he lifts her hips and enters her from behind in a standing position.

6. If you have a table with a quilt on it behind the screen, a good position is one with him lying on the table with her sitting astride, sideways to the audience.

Watching

In some societies, watching others make love is part of life – people gather round and witness the sexual initiation of a member of their community to celebrate his or her passage into adulthood. In our culture sex-watching is taboo, but our curiosity about how other couples behave in private is insatiable. Being a witness to intimate sex can be a powerfully moving and erotic experience that bears no comparison to watching polished professionals perform in a sex club. It can also serve to inspire and teach new moves that you can incorporate into your own sex life.

All done with mirrors

Self-conscious? Try watching yourself with your partner in a mirror first. Communicating indirectly through your reflections can be an erotic experience in itself. In Afghanistan and Pakistan, betrothed couples get their first glimpse of each other in reflection. The pair enter the room through doors in one wall and their eyes meet in the mirror on the opposite wall. The belief is that the mirror shows them to each other as they will appear in Paradise.

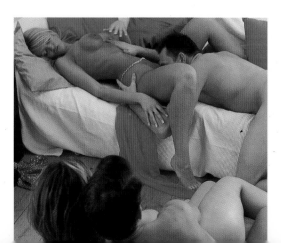

How to watch

1. Discuss the scenario fully with your partner. You may find that talking about it is enough...

2. If you decide to go ahead, choose your playmates carefully so that attraction between the couples is mutual and balanced. Beware of jealousy – if your partner is suspicious of your motives, don't do it!

3. Consider a threesome. Women are more likely than men to agree to a same-sex pairing and most men find the thought of their partner making love with another woman highly erotic.

4. Decide on your seduction tactics – maybe the woman in your partnership broaches the idea to her opposite number over a drink. If it's done right, even a refusal will boost everyone's ego, as it's flattering to think of two people lusting after you.

5. If the answer is yes, meet up in a relaxing setting to test the water – moving suddenly from friendship to sex-watching is bound to make you feel awkward.

6. Talk about what you'd like to do and set limits, such as watching only – no touching!

7. Prepare a seductive and non-threatening setting, with lots of drapes, cushions and candles. Offer your visitors use of your bathroom and sarongs or robes until they are ready to undress. Turn the lights down low, put on soft music, open the wine and relax into the experience...

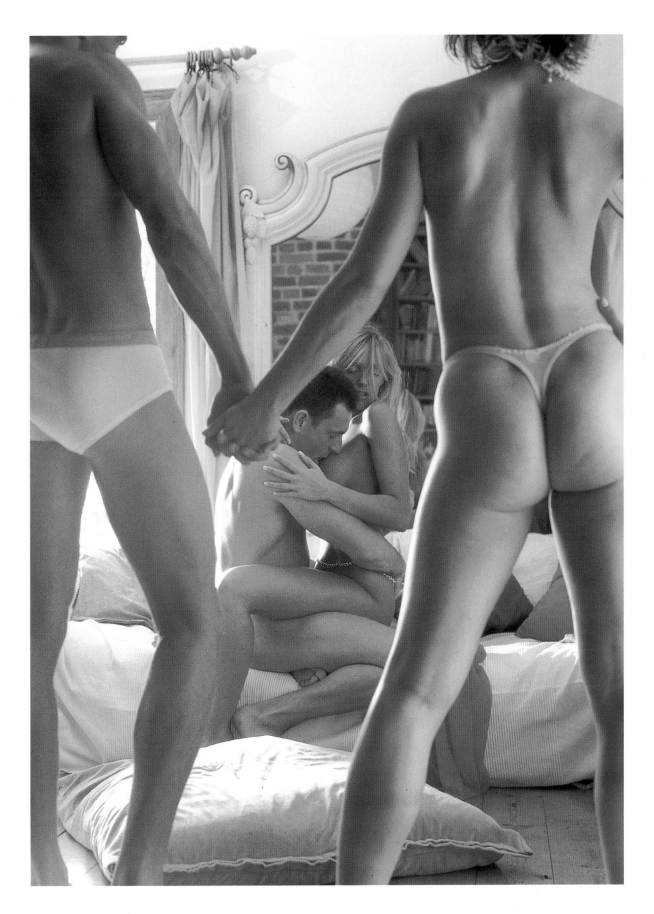

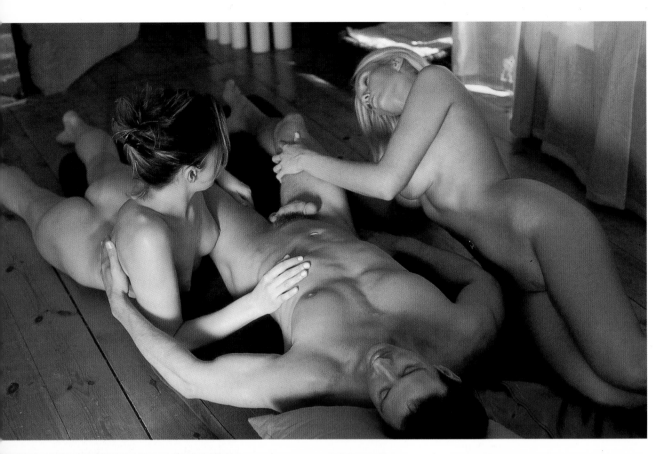

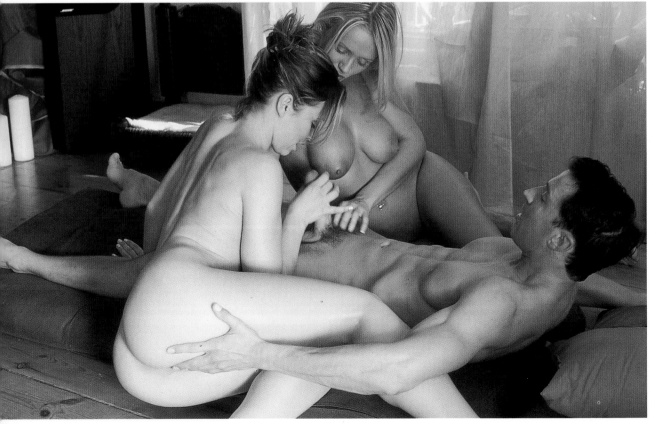

Massage for him

This is a sophisticated sexual treat to give, but only when you feel no jealousy. You can be sure your generosity will be well rewarded. In the middle of his birthday party, take your partner upstairs to your bedroom, promising that a surprise present awaits him. Outside the door, cover his eyes with a mask. Once you are inside, lock the door. Unseen by him, two or three of your female friends are waiting...

The Surprise

Suddenly he feels many hands gently undressing him. Still blindfolded, he lies down on a quilt or soft mat on the floor. You and your friends surround him and to seductive music simultaneously begin to massage his naked body with aromatic oils. This delicious experience reaches a climax in a many-handed erotic massage.

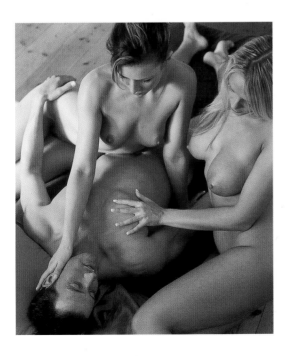

The six-handed massage

Begin with the lucky recipient lying on his front.

The first person starts by massaging his neck and shoulders, working gently to ease knots of tension.

The second person devotes herself to his back, loosening tension between the ribs with a circular pressure of the fingers, then walking her thumbs firmly down either side of his spine from top to bottom.

While the first person moves on to the arms, working her way down to the fingertips, pulling, shaking gently, and releasing them, the third person performs a similar massage on the legs, ending with the toes.

The second person meanwhile has reached the buttocks, which she kneads firmly and lifts provocatively.

It is now time for the recipient to turn over.

As before, the first person works on the sides of the neck and the shoulders, later moving on to the arms and hands.

The second person works on the torso.

The third person works on the legs, right down to the feet.

With the recipient well aroused, the second person moves on to the genitals. It is up to you how many of you share this task – it depends how generous you feel!

Massage for her

This is the ultimate gift from a man who is secure in his love. Draw your partner a deliciously deep bath scented with exotic perfume and pour her a drink. Once she is relaxed, explain that she must put on a blindfold and should trust you that the experience you are about to give her will be one of the most exquisite of her life.

Gentle treatment

Soap her body gently, then lift her out of the bath and pat her dry. Carry her to your bedroom and lay her down on a soft quilt on the floor. Unseen by her, two of your friends are waiting. The three of you surround her and begin to give her a deeply relaxing massage that culminates in the ultimate erotic experience.

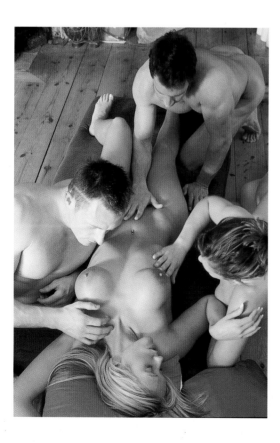

Massage with six hands and three tongues

Start with the recipient lying on her front.

The first person attends to the neck and shoulders, teasing out any knots of tension.

The second person devotes himself to her back, loosening the ribcage with circular movements of the fingers, and walking his thumbs down the length of her spine at either side.

The third person works on the legs, gently massaging the muscles of the thighs and calves.

While the first person works down the arms to the fingers, teasing them, stretching them, dropping them, and the third person does the same with the toes, the second person kneads the buttocks with his hands, pulling them apart and teasing the crease between them with his tongue.

It is now time to turn her over.

The first person works on the neck, shoulders and arms.

The second person works on the abdomen and hips.

The third person works on the legs and feet.

When she is fully ready, the third person pushes her legs up and out so they are splayed with her feet on the ground. Then he and the first person take their positions at either side of her and hold her legs in position. The second person moves between her legs. While he cups her buttocks in his hands and gently licks her vulva and clitoris, the other two suck and lick her nipples.

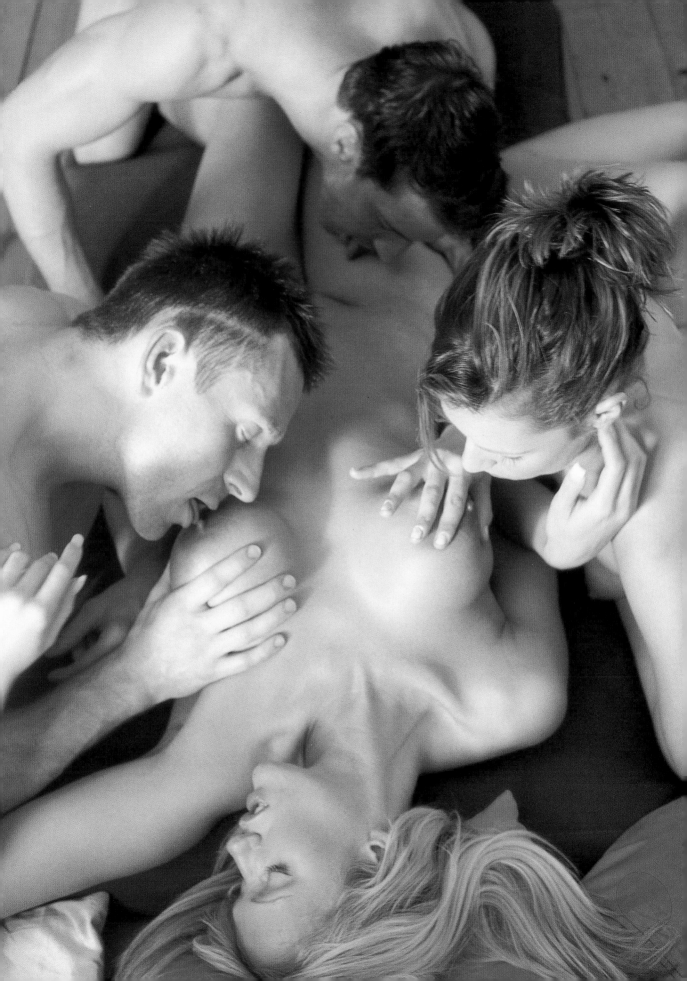

INDEX